— THE —
Big Silence

— THE —
Big Silence

A Daughter's Memoir *of* Mental Illness and Healing

KARENA DAWN

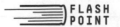

FLASH POINT

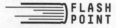 FLASH POINT

Published by Flashpoint™ Books, Seattle
www.flashpointbooks.com

Produced by Girl Friday Productions

Cover design: Emily Weigel
Production editorial: Tiffany Taing
Project management: Reshma Kooner

Image credits: front cover and flap photo © Nick Onken, back cover courtesy of the author

ISBN (hardcover): 978-1-954854-49-9
ISBN (e-book): 978-1-954854-50-5

Library of Congress Number: 2022900322

First edition
Printed in Canada

CONTENTS

AUTHOR'S NOTE

Some incidents and dialogues are drawn from my imagination and are not to be construed as verbatim, even though they are all based on real characters, conversations, and events. Memories of my childhood are sparse. Perhaps hiding my memories was a way to protect myself. So, to write this book, I have compiled my story from personal journals and poems, my sister Rachel's lyrics and poems, stories and song lyrics by my father, and my mom's stories. I have credited my family whenever I've included their poetry, journal entries, or songs, and have received permission for them to be included in this memoir. The flashbacks, memories involving conversations with other family members, songs, poems, essays, and journal entries from my childhood are italicized to differentiate them from the narrative.

Some places and many people's names have been changed, along with some features and characteristics, to preserve their anonymity.

The emotions, the pain, the despair, the love, the hope, and the story are all real.

PROLOGUE

Homeless.

The woman hunched over the garbage can at the corner of a rest stop in Turkey Run State Park. Rummaging for something to eat, she pulled out discarded bags of fast food and found some cold, wilted french fries. Now and then, she'd find part of a hamburger that had been thrown away. Her eyes darting all around to see if anyone was watching, she gobbled down a leftover sandwich, licking her dirty fingers afterward.

She was surely homeless. No one with a home would be that dirty. Or that hungry. Any passerby could see that her skin was hidden behind layers of grime and her hair hung like a tangled mop of brown, with long, straggly strings dangling over her shoulders. She wore a torn oversized sweater—not nearly thick enough to keep her warm on nights that dipped to near zero—jeans that were several sizes too big, and a pair of mismatched hiking boots that probably came out of a dumpster, like her meal.

A man driving by didn't know what to do. Should he report her? He slowly pulled his car alongside the woman and rolled down his window. "Hello! Hello! Is there anything I can do for you?"

She whipped around as if she had been stung. The man was surprised too. What he saw was a face that looked much younger than she'd seemed, and underneath that mop of dirty brown hair were shockingly bright and blue eyes.

—

This was my mother. A homeless person who ate out of garbage cans. Who had disappeared from our home and left me, my sister, and my father because she thought we were corrupted by Satan.

Time after time, we tried to help her escape the voices in her head. We tried to prevent her from running away from home and becoming homeless. I felt her guilt, her helplessness, and her desperate cries. I felt her frustration, her fear. There was so little I could do. Or that my sister could do. Or my father. Or my relatives. But we all tried.

It seemed that Mom always gave in, letting the illness take control. When I was younger, I thought she could fight back and was angry because I didn't think she tried hard enough. For us as a family. But as I have grown, I've learned that mental illness is a powerful adversary and one of the most difficult challenges a person can ever endure. Not everyone succeeds in fighting back.

After trying to make things right and help my mother, I learned how to surrender to the fact of her illness and work to make my own life better. I also watched my father rise above it all. I tried to do the same, but in my youth, I wasn't always successful. Dad wasn't perfect, but I saw his faith and enormous strength, and, in time, that helped me overcome my anger and all the hardships so I could move forward.

Mom's illness chiseled the skin off my bones until I was raw and ragged, but it helped shape me into the person I am today, and I am grateful for that. None of us is born a victim. We all endure grief and suffering in this life. No matter who you are, or how privileged, no matter the color of your skin or ethnicity, we all are faced with hardships. No one escapes this fact. When you realize that moments of suffering can be a gift, it will change you. Suffering teaches us to dig deep and find that inner core of courage, strength, and determination to move onward. To learn from the lessons and turn them into golden opportunities. You can be the hero of your own destiny. You can be the creator of your dreams, which can lead you to success in your career, relationships, and in love.

We all have a spark of greatness deep down within us. It's up to each and every one of us to uncover that greatness and become the better versions of ourselves. Not that it's always easy; it's not. And many people find it more comfortable to give up or blame someone else. But you don't have to do that. You can recognize that the pain and suffering are fine-tuning you and making you a better person.

Like everyone, I am a work in progress, and that's OK. I continually learn from my experiences, my mistakes, and my successes.

This is my story, but it's also my mother's because it's impossible to write mine without telling hers too. Her illness is a part of me. It is a part of my father, my sister—my family. It has been present in my daily thoughts as my biggest worry and also my biggest hope. It is the source of my strength and my fears, and it has formed the foundation of my present and future.

Moreover, this is my story about growing up with a mother who abandoned me. About a mother who has been mentally ill with schizophrenia and how that affected my world. But the beautiful thing about this story is how my family and I have overcome the most difficult misfortunes and discovered the most exquisite gifts in life.

If, by telling this tale, I can inspire other women and men to take their pain, tribulations, and failures and turn them into happiness and success . . . if I can motivate others to dig deep and dream about a better life, and then act on that dream, then I have done my job. We are all *more—brighter* and *stronger*—than we could have ever imagined.

It is my goal to serve as a beacon of hope and inspiration, guiding you on your own unique path in life.

To dream, to hope, to love—what could be better?

—Karena Dawn

"I FORGOT HOW TO PRAY"

Lyrics by Rachel Sahaidachny
Song by Nick Ivanovich

For a while I forgot how to pray
Every morning I woke up vacant
To gray light seeping through the shades

And now when I look back
Every bone in my neck cracks
What was I searching for?
I wonder who I am looking for

I've got my hand on the door in front of me
My fingers tremble as I turn the key

When I depend on someone
Can I depend on me?
Every side is sliding

I dreamed I drove into the river
But my car didn't sink
I had someone I loved beside me
And the car didn't sink
We careened wildly on the water
Crashing through the currents
Skidding over whirlpools
I was driving on the water
As if it were a road
But I was barely in control

I didn't sink
And neither did you

When every side is sliding
If I depend on someone
Can I depend on you?
Will you depend on me?

I've got my hand on the door in front of me
But my fingers tremble as I turn the key
Can I depend on me?

When every side is sliding
I always slip through

— THE —
Big Silence

PART ONE

Before the Sunset

CHAPTER ONE

"Kick the Dust Off Your Shoes"

Song and lyrics by Nick Ivanovich

At times, our best-laid plans
Are like houses built on shifting sand.
Fire and smoke may blacken the sun
But I know that Sunday will come.
And I bring good news.
Just kick the dust off your shoes
And move on.

I had no warning.

There is never a warning for these kinds of things. And yet I somehow knew that, at any moment, something could happen to change my world drastically, and when it did, I had to be ready to kick the dust off my shoes and just get moving. I was learning to pay attention to small things and big things. Impossible things. I was beginning to understand how everything connects like pieces of a puzzle and affects one moment to the next. Things like emails.

Generally, I got up before Bobby in the mornings. I loved the alone time so I could do yoga, meditate, paint on my easel, write in my journal, and plan my day.

On an October morning in 2016, just three months after my wedding to Bobby, my cell phone buzzed, alerting me that I had a new email message. I had been drifting in sleep, preparing to get up. For some reason, that morning, even before my cell phone buzzed, I wanted to lean over for a morning kiss. As if I wanted to seal that moment of perfect harmony in time. Of just him and me. Because our lives were not all perfect moments.

Bobby had reignited my creative imagination and ideas. A passion that I hadn't felt in a long time sprang to life after I met him. I was once again inspired to paint, dance, write poetry, and expand my business even more. I was now alive to the possibility of anything. And it was because Bobby supported me and inspired me to be freer, to be more me, to be more exciting, more adventurous, more powerful, and more alive.

The email was from my office assistant, Seth. *Your mother is in the hospital.*

My gut clenched.

Shit! Please, no!

I hadn't heard from my mother in quite some time, which was typical of our on-again, off-again relationship. I knew that she had recently found some stability in her life in Washington State, living in a rented cottage and holding down a job as a social worker. But her stability was always a fragile, temporary thing.

I threw off the covers and jumped out of bed.

"Fuck. Shit."

My heart lurched at the mention of my mother in the email. Fear. Worry. Disappointment. *What could be wrong?* Mom and I had not talked for several months, and I had no idea she was sick again. But I wasn't surprised. Not really. When your mom has a track record like my mother's and a history of schizophrenia, anything could happen.

"What's going on?" Bobby sat upright, stretching his arms and yawning.

"Mom's in the hospital. That's all I know right now. I have to call Seth at the office." He generally went into the office early.

"Oh, shit." Bobby knew this could mean anything when it came to my mother.

I called Seth, and when he answered the phone, I asked him, "What happened?"

"I don't know much. Your mom's friend Deborah sent a message to the office. You should contact her."

I had Deborah's phone number because I often called her to check on Mom. I quickly phoned her to find out what was going on.

"Karena, your mom had a stroke," she said. "She listed you as next of kin, so I wanted to make sure you knew about this."

Deborah's blunt tone scraped across my sleepy ears like a razor. My heart dropped. My mind raced with a thousand what-if thoughts. *Mom paralyzed. Mom in a wheelchair. Mom not able to feed herself. Mom not able to speak. Mom not able to go to the bathroom by herself.*

"Now, don't worry," Deborah hurried on. "She's not paralyzed or anything. And she can talk all right. I just thought you should know about it. I found your email on your Tone It Up website."

My Tone It Up business was all about health, fitness, and wellness, but at the time, I didn't see the irony of receiving such bad news through that platform. Right then, all I knew was that my mouth was dry. I needed water. Coffee. Something.

Deborah said that Mom had been in the hospital for four weeks already, and all the medical staff had been asking about her family. "At first Linda, I mean, your mom, wouldn't give them any family names."

Fuck. Shit. Hell. Dammit. Typical Mom.

I went into hyperdrive. I had to get to her and take care of things.

"Is she in Aberdeen?" I asked.

"No, she was in Aberdeen first, but they had to transfer her to a bigger hospital in Seattle because the one in Aberdeen was too small and they couldn't keep up with her blood transfusions. You know about those, right?"

Actually, I did not know about that. I knew about the ones she had when she was a teenager, but not about these current ones. I didn't want to talk to Deborah about how little Mom communicated with me.

"Yes," I lied. "I know about those."

"You're coming to visit her, right?"

"Of course," I said.

I slammed the phone down. "Shit, shit, shit!" I was furious that my mother had not called me.

"What's wrong?" said Bobby. "Karena, please calm down."

I paced the room. Early-morning sunshine was beginning to stream in golden rays through the bedroom window, ushering in the promise of a bright, wonderful day. Most days were like this in Manhattan Beach, California. But today was starkly different.

Skunk, our little Pomeranian butterball of black-and-white fur, bounced into the room, alerted to the fact that something was wrong. She looked up at me with solemn eyes, perhaps wondering if this was going to interfere with her breakfast.

"C'mon, talk to me," said Bobby, getting out of bed. "What happened?"

I explained what Deborah had just told me. "I can't believe Mom didn't call me." I shook my head in disbelief and ran my fingers through my hair. "I've got to call the hospital and find out what's happening."

My heart thudded fast and furious.

"I'll make you an espresso," said Bobby. "It's going to be OK. We'll figure this out."

He headed to the kitchen with Skunk following him, eager for her breakfast.

I called the hospital and spoke to one of Mom's nurses.

The nurse told me that, before Mom came to the hospital, she had been off work for two weeks, lying at home in bed, vomiting blood into water bottles. When her left arm went numb, she recognized that she had symptoms of a stroke and called 911 for help.

"Karena, your mom . . . um, *Miss Linda*," the nurse explained, "she has no friends to help her, no one to turn to. The first few days, she wasn't able to move her left arm, but she now has full use of it."

Miss Linda. Yes, that was my mother. I could sense that the nurse was blaming me for not being there. In her eyes, that made me the *worst* kind of daughter. Which was wrong. All wrong. But I didn't have time to explain to the nurse my history with Mom.

"So, she's going to be OK?" I asked, chewing on my bottom lip.

"We think so," the nurse said. "We just need to find a place for her to go right now on a temporary basis. Maybe a nursing home. We need the hospital bed for other patients, and there's nothing more we can do for her here."

"Don't do anything," I said. "I'm flying out first thing tomorrow, and I'll take care of everything." This was my usual reaction in intense situations. "Right now, please transfer me to Mom's room."

"OK," the nurse said.

Impatiently, I waited.

The phone rang several times.

"Hello." The voice was faint. Weak. But unmistakably, it was my mother.

"Mom? This is Karena." I was shaking, I was so angry at Mom. Just hearing her voice made me nervous. Anxious.

"Oh . . . hi, Karena."

She laughed in that strange way that bordered on condescension and nervousness. No excitement. No warmth. But I could tell she was surprised to hear from me.

"What's going on, Mom?"

"How did you know I was in the hospital?" she asked.

"Your friend Deborah."

"Oh."

"Mom. Are you all right?"

"I had a stroke . . . but I'm fine now."

She was being very vague, not giving me any details.

"Why didn't you call me?" I asked.

"It was no big deal."

"But you've been there for four weeks! That is a big deal. What's going on?"

"I'm losing two to four pints of blood per week, and they've been doing tests to see what's wrong. They say I have many health issues."

"I'll figure something out," I said. "Don't let them move you anywhere, though. I'll take care of this."

I decided I'd wait until I arrived in Seattle before letting her know I was there, worried that she might disappear from the hospital if she knew I was coming.

I hung up the phone and went to the kitchen for that espresso.

It was only a year and a half before this moment that Mom had become homeless for what felt like the millionth time, according to Aunt Carol, Mom's sister. There had been times when she wasn't homeless, though. Earlier, she had gone to Naples, Florida, to take care of her mother when she got sick; Mom was there until my grandmother died.

Mom then searched the Internet to find areas of the country that she might enjoy, and believed that Hood River, Oregon, would be an ideal new home. By 2014, she had saved money, quit her stable job in Florida, and driven west. Along the way, she stopped and visited me and Bobby in our home in Manhattan Beach. We were engaged to be married at the time, and her staying with us caused some turbulence in our relationship. That was the last time I'd seen her.

When Mom stayed with us in Manhattan Beach, we gave her the guest room so she could have privacy. But she didn't stay inside the house for very long. It was typical of her to disappear for hours at a time. I always wondered what she was doing. I thought that she was probably drinking in secret, which reminded me of my troubled childhood and all the times she had disappeared. Mom had abandoned me, my sister, and Dad long ago. Mom left us time and time again at home in Indianapolis. Rachel, my older sister, wanted nothing to do with me and escaped by hanging out with her friends all the time. Dad detached by playing guitar and performing in cafés and bars, staying out all night long. I was alone most of the time. Trying to be an adult. I had created a shell, a facade to protect myself from the pain that festered deep in my soul. That shell was still present, and because of this, I sometimes locked my husband out. Not a good thing. I knew I had to work on this or it would destroy our marriage. I was still dealing with abandonment issues. Only recently had I started talking to a therapist about my trauma.

Now I was stressed and worried that Mom would want to live with me and Bobby on a permanent basis. *How could I take care of her?* I wasn't equipped to be a caregiver. I was in my early thirties, managing my crazy, hectic work schedule, and I was hardly an expert at caregiving, even though it felt like I had been doing it in one fashion or another for a long, long time. Actually, I became the parent to my mother when I was only eleven or twelve years old.

I needed coffee. *Strong* coffee. The aroma of a fresh-brewed espresso wafted through the hallway as I made my way to the kitchen. Yes, I wanted *coffee*. I wanted *espresso*. And lots of it. Normally, I would have been hungry and could have whipped up some protein pancakes. But right now, my stomach was too knotted up to think about food.

Bobby had an espresso ready for me. Skunk sat on the floor,

finishing her breakfast and staring out the glass doors, watching a bird that had just perched on our patio.

"Thanks." I inhaled the aroma, blew on it to cool it, and took a big gulp. The hot liquid scorched my throat, but I didn't mind.

I sat down at the breakfast table. I knew we had to talk about Mom and her condition.

"What are you going to do?" asked Bobby.

"I'm not sure," I said. "First thing I have to do is fly to Seattle right away—she has no one else to help her—and I need to make sure she has a place to stay once they release her from the hospital. I don't think she can go home and live by herself." I held my cup with both hands as if I were hanging on for dear life, and took another sip.

"Karena, you know that I care, and I'm not being mean here, but we're not equipped to take care of your mom and all the drama that follows every time she's in our house." Bobby looked at me with a plea in his eyes, his hands folded around his own cup.

"I know," I said before he could continue. "It wouldn't be a good situation with all of Mom's problems."

"It's just that I feel angry at your mom for all the times she left you and cut you out of her life. Her actions are like a broken record. They just repeated with her drama concerning our wedding. It never changes with her, and I don't want to see her hurt you again." The drama with our wedding was just the most recent in a long list of conflicts with my mom.

"I promise you, Bobby, she won't have to live with us. I won't let her hurt me again. I'll figure out something."

But I knew he was worried. And so was I. Bobby was patient and kind, but even he had limits.

"I'll go with you to Seattle," Bobby said finally.

I shook my head. "No, this is my problem and I'll take care of it. You've got too much going on with your business. We can't both take time away."

"No. I'm coming with you." He could be stubborn. "I'll just move around some appointments on my schedule. It's no problem, and Julie will look after Skunk." He was right: our neighbor Julie was always willing to watch our dog.

"Are you sure you want to come?" I asked. I didn't like the idea of burdening him with this. I had already asked so much of him. And yet, having him with me would be a great comfort.

"Of course. It'll be all right, Karena." He reached over the table, took one of my hands, and held it. He had strong hands with callouses that could fix anything, except this. Strong hands that held my feelings, hopes, and dreams.

Frankly, I didn't know what I had done to deserve Bobby, but I was grateful. I knew that working through these issues with my mom wasn't easy for him.

I called Rachel, then Aunt Carol and Uncle Bill, and told them what had happened. They all promised to visit Mom in the hospital the first chance they got. I seemed to be the only one panicking.

She could be dying, the nurse told me, I kept thinking to myself over and over.

Bobby and I booked a flight from California to Seattle for the next day. For a moment, I could pretend that we were just a young couple going off on an adventure somewhere. We often traveled, and it could have been simply another flight to an island or New York or Montreal. But unfortunately, it was a journey into the unknown, where I would encounter the onslaught of emotions that I often tried to protect myself from and even ignore. Fear. Resentment. Hope. Love.

I moved into autopilot as I prepared for the trip. My hyperactive state slowed down, and I tried to be invisible and disappear within myself so I could be alone and process everything that was happening.

I wasn't sure what I was going to have to do once I arrived in Seattle, but it felt as though my life was going through a huge transition. And in that transition, there was a lot of fear.

—

"I'm not going to eat that," I say defiantly, staring at a plate of bland sautéed tofu. "You can't make me eat that." I have been sitting here for fifteen minutes at the kitchen table while Momma stomps around the room with an angry look on her face. Rachel has already eaten hers and was allowed to leave the table. Momma won't let me go until I eat that awful stuff. She wants me and Rachel to eat healthy, but some of the food is just not good.

"We'll see about that," Momma says. "You can't talk back to me like that, Karena!" She begins hitting my arm with a spoon. My arm is just a skinny thing of bones.

"Ouch! What are you doing, Momma?" I back my chair away from her, but she continues her onslaught, moving toward me, snapping that spoon on my arm until welts appear.

She repeatedly hits me until my arm stings and I start crying.

"No!" I shout at her. "I'm not hungry."

"I'll teach you not to talk back to me! You're only seven years old, and you think you can sass me like that!"

I turn from her and run out of the kitchen and up the stairs. On the landing, I sit down and look through the rails of the stairway. Momma is always mad these days, it seems. Sometimes she will be in a good mood and even throw pretend birthday parties for me. I like those times. I can dress up for my parties, and Momma will play the Beatles on the record player and serve my friends cake and ice cream. And often, Momma lets me play alone in our basement. I like being alone, and I build furniture out of cardboard and cover it with blankets. Sometimes I create caves with the blankets and invite imaginary friends over. Once in a while, I can have real friends over to crawl through the caves. And Momma leaves us alone.

Momma stands there at the bottom of the stairs, smacking the spoon on the palm of her hand, eyes wild as she rants. "I wish I never had you, Karena. Do you hear me? You were a mistake."

I get up from the landing and run into my bedroom and close the door, crying.

—

As a child and into my teenage years, my defiance became my resilience and strength. It was my fuel. My energy. It kept me alive. It would now have to keep me alive, once again.

CHAPTER TWO

Broken Soul

"Waiting for You"
Song and lyrics by Nick Ivanovich

Seasons change.
There's a time and a purpose for everything.
But look at you and me.
And the joy a new day can bring.

Drool.

It dribbled out the corner of my mouth and down my chin.

I opened my eyes.

"Did you have a good nap?" Bobby asked, glancing sideways at me.

"I think so," I said, wiping my mouth. "I dreamed about when I was a little girl."

"A good dream or bad dream?"

"An OK dream about defiance." I tried to smile.

He leaned in closer. "You OK, Kar?"

"Yes." I grabbed my purse from under the seat in front of me, pulled out a tissue, and wiped the drool from my chin.

"I didn't want to wake you when they served breakfast and coffee," he said. "I figured you needed the rest. I know you didn't sleep much last night."

"Thanks," I said. "We can pick up something on the road."

The last thing I remembered after the plane took off from LAX was guzzling down a mimosa, then closing my eyes. The two passengers in the seat across the aisle were talking about business meetings and sales forecasts and droned on and on about profitability ratios. I wanted to scream at them to shut up. That there were more important things than sales and profitability ratios. But I said nothing.

I continued to worry about Mom. *What would she be like in the hospital? Would she be the loving mother she could be when I was a little girl, or would she be the paranoid religious zealot / conspiracy theorist who believed we were all going to hell?* The grief I experienced from Mom's illness had stayed with me since I was very young. There were many moods, movements, colors, shapes, and textures to this grief, and it took me below the surface where, if I wasn't careful, I might drown.

It had been a three-hour flight from LA to Sea-Tac. Gratefully, I had finally relaxed and was able to get some rest. Now, the overhead seat-belt sign dinged and lit up. Bobby and I both lifted our trays and locked them into an upright position. As we began our descent, miles and miles of green mountains and hillsides sailed beneath us.

After we landed and collected our luggage, we rented a car, picked up Starbucks coffees and muffins, then headed to the W Seattle hotel downtown, where I'd booked a suite.

As we drove, Bobby and I made small talk, avoiding the question of what we would do about Mom.

The city sidewalks teemed with people. I had always associated Seattle with three things—Starbucks, music, and hippies—and the city was indeed filled with coffee shops on every street and musicians entertaining on the sidewalks with their guitars. But because of the *reason* we were there, the lively atmosphere didn't feel special.

Our hotel room wasn't ready when we arrived, so we headed next door for more Starbucks coffee. Outside, it was a gray day, and as we sat near the window, I drank my coffee quietly and noticed an elderly couple slowly strolling along the sidewalk, shuffling their feet through the wet leaves, arm in arm. Now and then, they smiled and paused to watch a squirrel scamper by or a brown sparrow swoop down from a tree branch to feed on seeds that had been scattered by other passersby. The couple didn't seem to mind the slight wind chilling the air or the threat of rain in the charcoal sky. Instead, they were absorbed in conversation with each other.

I was humbled. And a little wistful. I could imagine that they had lived a long, happy life together, filled with many family get-togethers where they were surrounded by children and grandchildren. My family was not that kind of family, although it had started out that way.

"They seem really happy," I mentioned to Bobby.

"You never know, Karena," he said. "They may be happy now, but they might have had a lot of heartache in their lives. Everyone has rough times."

"You're right," I said. "I tend to fantasize sometimes that other families are perfect, and yet I know that's not true. Every family has broken times . . . broken pieces in their lives to some extent. Everyone experiences pain. It's just how we manage it that makes the difference. We have to find a way to allow it to manifest into a blessing somehow."

"Speaking of *broken*, are you gonna call your mom and let her know we're here?"

"Yes. I have to, although I have no idea how she'll react."

Bobby nodded.

I called the hospital and told Mom that Bobby and I were in Seattle. If it was all right, we were coming to see her, I said. She didn't argue, but she didn't sound excited to see us either.

"She didn't hang up on me. So I guess that's a good sign," I told Bobby.

"I'm sure she'll be happy to see you, Kar. You're all she has, really." My sister, Rachel, had kept her distance from Mom since we were teenagers.

"I'm nervous about it," I said. "I have no idea what she's expecting of me. And, really, I have no idea just how bad she is or what kind of medicine she's on."

"We'll just take this one step at a time, OK?" Bobby finished his coffee. "Let's go back and see if our room is ready."

"Yeah, I want to get this visit over with."

When we finally checked into our suite, it was perfect. There was a living room with a lush, overstuffed sofa and a bedroom with floor-to-ceiling windows that offered panoramic views of Puget Sound. There was simply every amenity one could imagine. A wet bar with a refrigerator, wineglasses, and ice buckets. Gigantic soft towels and bathrobes. A surround-sound flat-screen TV and music system.

Bobby particularly liked the Jacuzzi next to the picture window. And I loved the double bathtub, which was similar to the Roman tub we had at home where Bobby and I often took bubble baths together. There was also a massive glass-walled shower in the bath. Bobby thought I was being extravagant, but I explained that I had booked this suite because I believed we would need a place that could offer us beauty, peace, and sanctuary after visiting Mom. I knew that visiting her would be difficult, challenging, and even heartbreaking.

After we unpacked, Bobby and I freshened up, threw on sweaters and jackets, and left our suite. I just wanted to make it to the hospital and get this over with. I had to learn exactly what was going on with my mother and then figure out what I was going to do about the situation. There would be no easy answers.

Once we reached the hospital, we parked in a visitor parking space and got out of the car. The autumn air was brisk, and a few leaves tumbled across the parking lot, which was wet from rain the previous night. Seasons change, and with those changes, life fluctuates from good to bad, bad to good, and everything in between. This was a moment of in-between, and somehow I would have to find the positive in all of this.

I pulled my jacket snug around me. The wind felt cold. Bobby took my hand as we walked in silence to the hospital's entrance. Inside, the sterile hallway with its polished floors led us toward the elevator. Several people got on with us and started pushing buttons for their floors. I remembered that the nurse said Mom was on the fourth floor.

I hated hospitals. This was not the first time I'd visited my mother in one.

Bobby and I got off the elevator and headed down the hallway to find Mom. I was glad she was out of the ICU and in a regular room. That made me hopeful that she would live. I was trying hard to keep my emotions in check.

"I'll wait out here while you go inside," Bobby said when we reached her room. "If she wants to see me, I'll come in. Otherwise, I'll just be here waiting for you."

"All right. I'll see how she is and let you know."

Bobby squeezed my hand. I took a deep breath and opened the door.

When I entered her room, I saw that there were two beds. A woman lying in the first one appeared to be napping. Mom was in the bed farthest from the door, next to the window. She was sitting up, looking out the window, and hooked up to an IV and a tube connected to a heart monitor. A pulse oximeter was clamped on her finger.

Mom turned and looked at me.

It was always a shock when I saw her after we had not seen each other in a while. Her face was sunken and gray, and the wrinkled skin around her eyes seemed almost transparent, delicate as crepe paper. *Where was the beautiful goddess mother I had known when I was a little girl? The one who worked out to Jane Fonda and Kathy Smith VHS tapes and who became a vegetarian, eating only tofu and veggie burgers? The one who was obsessed with health when I was young?*

But I knew where *that* mother was. That beautiful goddess mother had disappeared long ago and had been taken away into a world of mental illness.

Now, Mom's body was small and frail, even though she was pudgy around the middle and a little overweight. Her frailty—and her illness—had consumed her. Long, wiry brown hair, streaked with gray and sorely in need of washing, framed her face. She was only in her early sixties. Far too young to look this decrepit and worn. But after the kind of life she had lived, I shouldn't have expected anything else.

When I was little, Mom sometimes reminded me of the actress Katharine Ross, who starred in the classic movies *Butch Cassidy and the Sundance Kid* and *The Graduate*. She had glistening chestnut-brown hair that curled on her shoulders and bright-blue eyes the color of the sky. Dad often talked about how pretty Mom was, and even after she got sick, he would tell her she was the prettiest woman in Indianapolis. I would often dress up in her clothes and put on her heels and red lipstick, thinking I looked like her. Like a movie star. Like a fitness model. Of course, that was *before* the illness ravaged her.

I had seen Mom off and on for years, and had witnessed the decline of her beauty, so I shouldn't have been surprised to see the way she looked in the hospital bed. But I always forgot in between our visits, and expected her to return to the woman she once had been.

I briefly recalled a novel that I'd read in college, *The Lover* by Marguerite Duras. In the story, the main character discusses her mother-daughter relationship and how it affects her throughout life, including her love affairs. The most obvious issues are caused by madness and depression. I understood that discourse on mother-daughter relationships. About mental illness, depression, hope, and love. It seemed like there was a thin line between madness and sanity in the real world.

Mom smiled. With dry and cracked lips, it was a sad smile and not the joyous ear-to-ear kind. "Hi, Karena. You came."

"Of course, I came. I told you I would when I called you."

I gave Mom a little hug, careful to not hurt her or interfere with the IV lines, and pulled up a chair to sit close by her bedside.

We talked a short while about everyday things: the weather, the food at the hospital, her social work job. And how she was doing, in general.

"I'm good, Karena."

"No, Mom, how are you doing, *really*?"

"They want to discharge me." Her face was deadpan. As if she had already figured everything out and there was nothing to discuss.

"But . . . but where? Where are they sending you?"

"I'm going back to Ocean Shores."

Ocean Shores was a small community along the Pacific coast of Washington. It was beautiful there, but there weren't many amenities. "Mom, you can't! The nurse told me you've been getting blood transfusions, and the closest place for blood transfusions is an hour away from Ocean Shores. And there's no cell reception in your house, so you can't even call a taxi!"

"I can drive. I have a car."

"Mom, you can't drive. You could pass out or any number of things." My voice sounded a little hysterical. *What were they thinking? They couldn't just put her on a bus and send her home!*

"I'll figure something out," I said. I paused and decided to pull in my support. "Mom, Bobby's here if you'd like to see him. He's waiting outside."

"Sure," she said. "I like Bobby."

I went to the door, stuck my head out, and called him in.

Bobby approached the bed. "Hi, Linda," he said.

"Hi, Bobby. I'm glad you came."

"How are you doing?" he asked as he pulled a second chair next to mine.

"I'm fine, really."

"That's good to hear," Bobby said.

The nurse came in to check Mom's vitals. She looked at us and nodded as if she approved of our visit. "It's good that you came," the nurse said.

I asked her about Mom's condition, and she told me the same information I'd been told on the phone.

"Your mother didn't suffer any long-term effects from the stroke. Her arm was numb for a couple of days, but she has full use of it now. But she has a bleeding disorder. We're not sure what's causing it."

I nodded, glancing from the nurse to Mom.

I still didn't know anything about Mom's *current* bleeding disorder. I knew Mom had this disorder when she was a young girl, and I had been told that it had stopped altogether when her father died. He had been an abusive man with schizophrenia and had died by suicide, and the doctors could not explain why her bleeding disorder stopped when it did. Evidently, Mom's bleeding started again later on in life after she was diagnosed with schizophrenia.

When the nurse finished checking on Mom, she looked pointedly at me. "Your mom needs you. It's good that you came," she repeated.

She nodded at me and Bobby as she left the room. We stood up to follow her.

"We'll be right back," I told Mom.

"OK." She turned her gaze to the window, her hands folded in her lap. She seemed to be surrendering to whatever was decided for her. Or maybe she was pretending. I wasn't sure.

"What's the plan for further treatment?" I asked the nurse out in the hallway.

"There's nothing more we can do for your mother. We need to

discharge her," she said. "Actually, Karena, we wanted to discharge her and send her home two weeks ago, but she needs biweekly blood transfusions and we're not sure if she can drive herself to get them or if she can even live by herself at this point. We didn't know who to call, and finally she gave your name as her next of kin. Then we were able to locate your mother's friend Deborah, who knew how to get in touch with you."

"You can't send her home!" I said. "She's not capable of living alone. Give me some time and let me figure out something."

"OK, but you need to find a place for her," the nurse said. "And soon."

"Shit," I mumbled quietly to Bobby before we returned to Mom's room.

I told Mom that her sister and her family would be there soon to visit too. I asked her if she was comfortable, and she said yes. After that, she didn't say much else, and I wasn't sure if my presence was appreciated or not.

"Mom, Bobby and I are here to help. I'm going to find a place for you to live."

Again, she didn't say anything. She looked down at the blanket's edge and started picking at it as if distracted.

"Do you want my help, or do you want me to leave?"

I never knew what Mom wanted from me, and I needed to know.

"No, I don't want you to leave," she said. Tears welled up in her eyes. "I want you to help me. You're all I have, Karena."

"All right," I said. "We'll go now, and Bobby and I will work with the doctors and find you an assisted-living place where you can go. Then we'll drive to Ocean Shores and clean out your cabin. You can't go home and stay by yourself."

"I'll be fine on my own in Ocean Shores," Mom said. "Just help me get out of here, OK?"

"No, you can't go until I find a place for you. You can't even drive in your condition, Mom, and you can't stay alone."

She seemed to surrender. Or maybe she was just too weak to argue. "Thanks."

I leaned over and hugged her.

My eyes filled with tears. How was it that I, a thirty-five-year-old daughter, was the caregiver now? How was it that I, the one who should be able to lean on her mother for advice and friendship, had become the adult while the mother had become the child once again? Part of me resented her for interfering with my perfectly organized life. But another part of me was heartbroken for all the loss, the hardships, and the illness, and I knew that I would do anything to help my mother. I loved her.

Mom had leaned on me for most of my life, even when I was little and, later, after she had left us. She would appear out of nowhere with her wild delusions and paranoia, ranting about a new religion or cult she had discovered, about our food and drink being poisoned by a secret government, or about dragons and monsters that lurked around every corner. She would pull me in and let me get close to her, and I would suck up all the love and attention I'd been denied, and then she'd disappear and abandon me. This happened time and time again.

Dad was no longer in her life. She left him officially when I was eighteen years old, but she had left all of us long before that, really.

"Bobby and I will be back, Mom, as soon as I get some things straightened out."

"OK, Karena," she said. "See you later."

Bobby and I walked quietly out of the hospital.

"She seems stable," he said.

"Yeah, for now. They have her on meds. But that stability won't last if she quits taking them."

We climbed into our rental and drove back to the W. We went out for dinner at an Italian café within walking distance, on the water's edge.

"We've got to find her a place to live," Bobby said finally. "She can't live with us."

"I know." My voice was low. I wanted to scream: *I know! I know! I know!*

Instead of screaming, I tried to be logical. "There has to be an assisted-living facility that will take her. I'll find a place, don't worry." But I *was* worried.

"OK. But I know how your mother is, and you have a lot on your plate already, Karena. I just don't want to see you get hurt. She's made you think she's OK before, then disappeared on you. This time, you're going to have to set some boundaries, you know. You can't let yourself become a martyr for her."

"Boundaries? Yes, you're right."

Mom tended to suck the air out of me, but if I could set boundaries, I'd be all right. I always had a hard time doing that. I had spent years suffering from the trauma of abandonment and Mom's illness, and yet I knew that this suffering had helped me to develop great strength, courage, and compassion for others. But I would drown if I didn't establish boundaries.

We walked back to the hotel, enjoying the fall evening air under a round orange moon like the ones I used to see when I was a girl in Indiana. The kind of moon that loomed over cornfields and hayfields and taunted us on Halloween nights. I hadn't seen that kind of moon in a long, long time.

The evening in Seattle was alive with energy—so different from the dreariness of the hospital. Musicians played their instruments on the sidewalks with their guitar cases open so we could toss in money to show our support. Couples, arm in arm, were strewn along the streets, on their way to restaurants or hotels, and basking in life.

I had long ago recognized that even though I was an introvert, I was a high-spirited person who thrived in an environment with music and dancing in the streets. I was not meant to live in dismal circumstances. I had always had dreams and desires and full-blown passions, even though, at times, I kept them to myself. Bobby said that I was caring, honest, hardworking, and generous to a fault. Most of all, he said, I was loving. I was an artist too, and adored painting and decorating my home and the homes that Bobby and I bought and refurbished.

I was beginning to understand that, as a *creative*, when I was asked to mother my own mother, I often reacted with depression, stress, and anger. That kind of demand can make a person feel used, unappreciated, consumed, and confined, not to mention almost nonsexual, because it strips away creative spirit and passion. Any relationship that drains creative reservoirs without the tenderness to refill them— which is what I experienced with Mom—was damaging to my psyche, my creativity, my sexuality. And it had nothing to do with how much I loved her. I loved Mom deeply. I wanted our relationship to be a normal mother-daughter one, and I wanted the best for her. I would swim across oceans for her. I would climb mountains for her. But I was doing the heavy lifting, trying to make this work, and Mom contributed very little. That's why I felt nearly drained by my mother's needs. From the "over-caretaking." Everything was overwhelming. There were so many things I had to tend to and manage. I felt exhausted.

I wasn't sure Bobby understood this, but he intuitively provided the love and care I craved. He allowed me to be myself. He let me be fiery and outspoken when I needed to express those energies. He let me be alone when I needed quiet. Bobby had nurtured a relationship that was responsive to both our creative and personal energies.

That night, after the visit to the hospital and dinner, Bobby and I tried to relax in our hotel. We opened a bottle of wine, and I lit candles and set them in various nooks and crannies around our suite. The candlelight cast a warm glow over the room and helped both of us settle down. We undressed and stepped into the Jacuzzi, sliding into the frothy water, letting the jets shoot and spray our bodies. The warm water soothed and massaged our sore muscles, and we sank lower into the water.

"Thank you, Bobby," I said.

"For what?" he asked, taking a sip of wine.

"For everything."

CHAPTER THREE

I Am Trying . . . but
I Am Not a Saint

So here we are again
Another chance to heal these wounds
Take my hand
I know you're afraid
But so am I
We are of the same flesh and blood
I believe we have the power
To heal each other.

—Karena, 2017

Caregivers are saintly people.

 I am not one of them. I am not a saint. I'm not a natural caregiver. But I'm trying my best. Don't get me wrong. I like taking care of people. I am nurturing. I am caring and loving. I try not to be resentful. I love to give to others in my personal life and in my professional life. Giving and being of service are everything to me. But stressful situations like ongoing caregiving can make life difficult. And sometimes it can be too much. Sometimes I feel like the "over-caretaker" who lacks the nurturing and regeneration time needed to restore my soul. If I am empty, I have nothing to give to anyone else.

The morning after seeing Mom at the hospital, I got up earlier than Bobby and went to the window overlooking Puget Sound. It was so quiet. The daylight cast a golden hue over the world, and for a moment, it restored some peace. It felt as if, in many ways, this journey was a kind of pilgrimage to discovering more about myself.

In the bathroom, I looked in the mirror. There were shadows under my eyes, which were filled with worry and anger, and a certain knowingness too. I didn't need to shout at my mother as I had in so many dreams. Instead, I had to act and speak my truth with honesty and courage and love. I had to live my life. And through my actions and courage, I had to resolve the issues with Mom's living conditions and, later, with our relationship.

I squared my shoulders and told myself I would be OK. Mom would be OK. My marriage would be OK. Right now, it was rough. Months later, Bobby and I would find our way to a therapist who focused on assisting couples through rough times in a marriage, which helped us find our way forward.

But in Seattle, Bobby and I had a long day ahead of us. I took a shower, then returned to the bedroom, where he was already up and packing our clothes. We had to get going.

"You all right, Karena?" Bobby had asked me this question a million times over the past couple of days.

"Yes, I just want to deal with this and get it over with."

"Me too."

We needed to head home, but first I called Mom and promised her that I would coordinate her care. Once we found her a place, I would come back to move her. Bobby promised he would help me move her out of the cabin in Ocean Shores.

"What more can I do to help?" he asked repeatedly.

"Nothing," I said. "I have to find the right place for Mom, and then figure out COBRA insurance, doctors, and transfusions for her. I'm sorry, but you can't really help. Just be patient with me, OK? I'll make this work."

"Karena, you're going to burn yourself out," he said. "You can't do everything on your own. Please let me help."

"It's all right," I said. "I'll take care of it."

Bobby was worried about me, but I had been taking care of things all my life. It's all I knew how to do. But now I was lucky to have him, my friends, and my business associates for support.

We left that day for California to take care of business. It was stressful back home. I wasn't able to relax. I couldn't focus on work, and I mostly stopped running and exercising. I also stopped doing yoga and meditating. And I shut Bobby out much of the time. I didn't mean to be cold or elusive, but I didn't want to burden him with my issues. A person can only take so much. One time, I joked that it was a good thing we got married *before* this crisis. Otherwise, he may have run the opposite way.

He just looked at me with sad eyes and hugged me. "Karena, we're in this together. I love you."

"I love you too." I broke down, crying in his arms.

—

I flew back and forth to Seattle from LA several times during the next few months to coordinate my mother's medical needs.

In January, Aunt Carol and Rachel came to visit Mom, who was still in the hospital (they had finally agreed to keep Mom until I could find a place for her to live). One morning, I met with Aunt Carol and Rachel for breakfast at the W hotel, where we had avocado toast with orange juice and espresso.

Rachel had not seen Mom in a long, long time. She had simply avoided Mom for years as a way to protect herself. I had long ago realized that Rachel's wounds from our childhood were so deep that they had been locked away. She painted and wrote poetry about the hardships while we were young but stayed away from home most of the time. She left for college two years ahead of me. Now she lived with her fiancé in Indianapolis, which made it difficult for us to visit often. But when we did get together, we immediately connected, taking comfort in one another because we fully understood the sadness of our childhood.

And yet, when it came to coordinating Mom's health care, there was no one to help me. Not really. It was frustrating and overwhelming.

"I'm going to see Mom again later today." Rachel sipped her orange juice.

"We can go together," said Aunt Carol. She turned to me. "You know, I want to apologize, Karena."

"For what?" I asked, nibbling at my toast.

"I was angry with you for a long time. I thought you'd abandoned your mother. I didn't fully understand that she was the one who left you kids. So when I told you that you needed to be a good daughter, I didn't know what I was talking about. So I . . . I . . . well, I apologize."

"That's OK," I said. "I understand."

"She always told me a different story," Aunt Carol said.

"She has a way of twisting things to make herself look good. She wants people to feel sorry for her," Rachel said, rolling her eyes.

"Aunt Carol, I always suspected Mom told you things that weren't true," I said. "And because you lived in Louisville, you couldn't actually see what was going on."

"Dad tried really hard to make up for Mom's shortcomings," Rachel said. "He was always telling Karena how beautiful and smart she was when she was little, and he was supportive of me, too, in his own way."

"Yes, your father tried his best," Aunt Carol said.

"But it wasn't perfect. Dad and I butted heads when I lived at home," I added. "Mom tried to get me to distrust him because of all her paranoia and delusions. A lot of the time, I was not very good to him. I admit that."

"You *were* rebellious. I remember that all too well," Rachel said. "You always did talk back to both Mom and Dad."

"You were rebellious too, Rachel, but quieter and sneakier about it," I said. "I was more openly defiant."

"Well, not to change the subject, girls, but we need to figure out a plan for your mom's finances," Aunt Carol said. "I don't think she'll be able to live on disability or social security."

Aunt Carol was a businesswoman and good with budgeting and finances. This was one way she could help out.

"Has your dad given your mom the money he owes her from the divorce all those years ago?" Aunt Carol looked first at Rachel and then at me.

"I don't know," both Rachel and I said at the same time, shrugging.

"Linda always said that your dad stole money from her, so it wouldn't surprise me if he withheld the divorce money."

"No, that's not true. She didn't even show up for the divorce proceedings," Rachel said. "She honestly didn't care at the time about any of that stuff. She just wanted her freedom and to be away from us."

"I don't think getting her money from the divorce is an option now," I said. "Mom was gone long before it was actually finalized. You already know that, Aunt Carol."

"That's right," Rachel said. "Mom abandoned the marriage and us kids even after Dad tried many times to make it work. He hung in there for a long, long time."

Neither Rachel nor I could figure out why our aunt was so focused on the divorce; it had been more than fifteen years since it was finalized.

"Well, your dad seemed to care more about playing music at some bar at night than being home with his family." Aunt Carol smirked. "If I remember correctly, he was out most nights, playing his music."

"Look, Mom was always welcome to go and listen to him play," I said. "She knew he was a musician when she married him, and at that time, she liked it and supported him. Besides, Aunt Carol, he was a good father to me and Rachel, even though he had his issues. There was a long time where we had our differences and butted heads, and I didn't like him very much. But he has always been there for us, and he still is. And I know he tried really hard to be a good husband to Mom. He took her back time and time again when she hurt him just as much as she hurt us."

"I agree with Karena," Rachel said, adding, "Dad was there for us when she wasn't."

Aunt Carol nodded. "Well, maybe you two can figure out how your mom can get by without a settlement from the divorce. I know it was a long time ago and probably a moot point right now. I'm not sure. I just know she won't be able to survive on a small social security check."

"I'll figure something out," I said.

There was clearly still a lot of tension and anger within the family. For many years, Mom had manipulated situations and people, trying to make me, Rachel, and Dad look like the "bad guys." She'd also made it seem like everyone was out to get her. But here we were for her, and it was good to talk through things and be with family while in Seattle.

We finished our breakfast and discussed what was happening in our lives other than Mom. But I was very worried about everything: Mom's finances, her health. What were we going to do? The conversation with Aunt Carol hadn't changed much; I knew it was mostly up to me to figure everything out.

After visiting Mom, Aunt Carol and Rachel would be heading to the airport to fly back home, so we said our goodbyes. They wished me luck with Mom and said to let them know if they could be of any help. I told them I appreciated their offer. Being in charge of Mom's situation was draining.

I sighed heavily and squared my shoulders. I wouldn't let it get me down. I had to stay strong. Tough. *I will persevere,* I told myself. *I have to be the caregiver.*

I gulped down the last of my coffee, paid my bill, and left the restaurant. I had work to do.

Before flying back to LA, I went to the hospital and talked to Mom about the various options I was researching. Then I leaned over to give her a small hug, and she whispered, "I love you."

What did she say?

I rose, shocked, then quickly regained my senses and whispered back, "I love you too."

Mom hadn't told me that she loved me since I was a little girl. Hearing it at this moment felt like a healing salve on a deep open wound.

I hurried out the door and fled to the bathroom and into the farthest stall. I leaned my head against the wall and sobbed.

—

Later, I wrote a letter to Mom, which I never gave her. It was a way to express my frustrations and feelings.

I AM STRONGER THAN YOUR CURSE

You're beautiful, Mom. That soul that lives deep behind your eyes and high above the sky. I love you . . . with the biggest heart a child could ever have. I looked up to you. I wanted to be as beautiful as you. I would even dress up in your clothes. Do you remember?

I cursed God when he took you from me and left me with an empty shell of what remains. I never truly got you back. You're sitting next to me, yes. But you're not here.

I want to grab you, shake you. Scream at you. Mom, I'M HERE! I'm HERE! Love me, teach me about life. Tell me your stories. I want to tell you mine.

Oh, how I can curse you and thank you in the same sentence. It's painful to hate yet only know how to love. There's an emptiness I carry. I know it must be you.

What happened? I was your little girl . . . You brought me into this world to love and teach and watch me grow. I still learned to love and grew in learning, but it was without you by my side, and that is my deepest sorrow.

I thank you, but at the same time I curse you. All these years I had to fight my way back up. Do you know this? I almost didn't make it!

But I am STRONGER THAN YOUR CURSE.

I am here.

So here we are again. Another chance to heal these wounds. Take my hand. I know you're afraid, but so am I. We are of the same flesh and blood. I believe we have the power to heal each other.

Just talk to me . . . let me inside your mind.

Tell me you're sorry. Do you know that for years I lived unable to love, to trust, to feel like I existed or mattered?

Tell me you're proud of me. For what I've overcome . . . for who I've become. Because it wasn't easy, but I did it.

How times have changed. When I needed you, you left me. But now you need me for survival. And I would never leave you like you left me.

I forgive you. I forgive you. I pray for you . . . your sweet lost soul. I believe you left a long time ago, but when I look for that mother who left a long time ago, I can feel your sweet love covering me from above.

Love,

Karena

CHAPTER FOUR

"We Don't Deal with Emotions"

"Salvation's Plan"
Song and lyrics by Nick Ivanovich

Sweet mysteries of life
Like the groom who finds his bride
Reconciled and justified
By the blood that flows through my veins tonight

I cannot comprehend
Your death for my sin.

Frustration.

I was not only frustrated but furious! How could it be so difficult to find a health-care facility that would take my mother? While I managed my Tone It Up business at home, I also searched for assisted-living places that would accept Mom. I couldn't find one. All of them said they weren't equipped to manage her blood transfusions, which she needed on a regular basis. Plus, they explained, "Her age is a factor, as well as her long list of medical and mental health conditions." Mom was only sixty-four, and that was young for these kinds of places.

I was frantic. I searched the Seattle and Aberdeen areas but could not find any help.

The hospital where Mom was staying needed to release her, but how could they when she couldn't live alone? I couldn't move to Washington and take care of her. And there was no one else in the world who would. And I wouldn't let them put her in a nursing home where she would surely languish.

Truth was, I hated this part of being a caretaker. It was exhausting. A thousand and one things had to be done. Whenever I found myself ruminating about this, I had to remember to just let go and surrender to love. I continually reminded myself that Mom had given me life. And because of Mom and all that she had done, that life was now beautiful and loving. Her mental illness had forced me to learn how to live on my own, how to build my dreams. I had learned how to let others love me and to allow myself to love and trust again. But it hadn't been easy. When I was younger, I believed her delusions. Fortunately, as I grew up, I realized it was her illness speaking.

I had to admit, however, that being charged with taking care of Mom's needs provided a way for me to liberate myself. To find my own salvation in this painful situation.

I talked to numerous doctors at the hospital about Mom's condition, explaining to them her history of mental illness. The doctors didn't seem interested. They told me they treated Mom for her stroke and other serious health issues and that these things were stable now. "We're giving her Prozac, and it's helping to stabilize her moods," one doctor said.

So, according to them, she had to be released. "We have other patients who need her bed," one doctor said. "We can do nothing more for her."

Where she went now did not matter to them. It was out of their hands. I had insisted on getting a psychological evaluation for Mom, but they had refused. One doctor actually said, "We don't deal with emotions here."

"You don't deal with *emotions*?" I snapped back. "Mental illness is *not* an emotional issue. It's a real disease. My mother is not mentally and physically able to survive on her own. That is a real legal issue, and as her physician, you're liable for that. And you should know that emotions don't come into play here unless there are suicidal tendencies and severe depression."

"Like I said"—the doctor smirked, ignoring everything I had just said—"we don't deal with emotions, and we've done all we can to help her here. It's time for her to go."

I was horrified at the doctors' responses and their detachment. They didn't seem to understand the holistic connection between mental and physical health. The more I thought about it, the more outraged I became. I was beside myself. The clock was ticking, and they planned to release her any day now. They presumed I would take her back to California and that would be the end of the story. I worried it could be the end of my marriage to Bobby. That it could ruin my business. I was *not* Superwoman! Didn't the doctors know this? Hell, they didn't care.

The doctors made it very clear that they were done with my mother. And they had no interest in how this would affect my life.

I tried to imagine Mom in our spare bedroom, sitting for hours by the window, occasionally coming out of her room to explain to us how the Antichrist was taking over the world and coming for us. She had done that before. I tried to imagine her sneaking out of the house and wandering down to the beach with a bottle of vodka in her hand, staring out at the horizon while telling anyone who would listen about the Antichrist.

Hell.

Hell!

I wanted to scream!

It was all too scary to think about. And there were so many other things to address besides where she would live. I insisted that Mom call her place of employment to tell them she wouldn't be back. There was no way she could be employed as a social worker any longer given her health conditions. And besides, how could she take care of anyone else's welfare when she couldn't take care of herself? I was also finally able to get Mom signed up for federal disability after many phone calls. That wasn't much of a monthly stipend, but it was better than nothing.

Every day, I contacted case managers and social workers and pleaded with them to work with me to keep Mom in the hospital until

I could find an assisted-living facility that would agree to take her. Sadly, they could not, and would not, offer me much help.

The physician who treated Mom's stroke told me, "You're going to have to take care of her, Karena."

"It's not practical or possible." I shook my head vehemently.

His voice was judgmental. "Your mother told the staff that her daughters didn't care about her. She said that they never visited her . . . and frankly, you should be ashamed of yourself. You should be a better daughter."

What?

I was stunned.

Speechless.

Furious.

"That is simply *not true!*" I screamed. I was at my wit's end. What kind of health-care system did we have in America? When did it become all right for a physician to shame a member of the patient's family? I couldn't believe that I was being called a bad daughter when, at the same time, he was telling me that his job as her doctor was done. I also couldn't believe Mom had told them that I never came to see her when I had tried for weeks and months to contact her before her stroke.

When I called Bobby, I ranted. I was so angry. So frustrated.

It all felt so hopeless. My life felt hopeless.

"Don't worry," Bobby continually said. "You'll find the right place for her."

But I knew he was beginning to doubt that I would. And with those doubts came worries about what would happen if I had to bring her home with me. I worried—I *knew*—that it would ruin our marriage.

I couldn't give up. *I am strong,* I told myself. I persisted with every ounce of energy I had.

I contacted the legal department at the hospital and reported the doctor who had shamed me. I also reported the doctor who had said that they didn't deal with emotions there. There was no excuse for this kind of treatment or attitude. I asked the hospital's legal team about whether I had any recourse. It was the last resort, but thankfully, it bought me some time.

After a while, I realized that it would be much easier to bring Mom to a facility near me in California where I could more closely monitor her care. Bobby thought that was a good idea too. "It will take a lot of stress off your shoulders. All this flying back and forth to Washington is taking its toll."

So I began to research facilities in California. Again, many places refused to take Mom because of her health history, age, mental illness, and her need for biweekly blood transfusions. They simply weren't equipped to handle her medical conditions, especially the blood transfusions.

I didn't know how much longer I could go on. By now, Mom had been in the hospital for more than three months.

Then I experienced a miracle. The hospital in Washington kept Mom for another three weeks, and I finally found her a lovely assisted-living home in Palm Springs, which was an easy driving distance from my house.

I was so overjoyed and relieved that I broke down and wept. Actually, I cried my heart out. But I also wanted to dance for joy. I wanted to run out to the beach and throw myself into the ocean waves and drift for hours and hours. I wanted to sing and twirl and laugh. I wanted to fly high into the starry sky and soar even higher into the cosmos. I was so happy. And Bobby was happy too.

He breathed a sigh of relief when I told him the good news.

"This will work out great for your mom and for us," he said.

That night, for the first time in a long while, after curling myself into Bobby's arms, I made love to my husband.

CHAPTER FIVE

"The Hellhole of the Pacific"

"Salvation's Plan"
Song and lyrics by Nick Ivanovich

As daylight kicks through the darkness
All the demons are put to rest.
The song of songs keeps playing in my head
Resurrecting me from the dead.

I'm here!

I want to grab you, Mom, shake you. Scream at you. I'm here. Love me. Teach me about life. Tell me your stories. I want to tell you mine! I am the child, remember? You've missed so much of my life, Mom!

—

Bobby and I were in the W hotel in Seattle again. We had taken the first flight available after learning that I could transfer Mom to the facility in Palm Springs. He had come to help me clean out her cabin in Ocean Shores and coordinate the move. Mom certainly would not be going back there.

I had been on cloud nine ever since I learned we had found a place for Mom, but that morning, I woke up feeling angry. In a dream, I had been shouting and screaming at my mother, begging her to listen to me. Begging her to be my mother. *I am the child, remember?*

I still had a lot of anger pent up inside. I had always been chasing after Mom's love. No matter what I did, no matter how hard I tried. Even now, I still felt like the abandoned little girl, and I still hoped that, in time, that feeling would finally go away.

Mom was diagnosed with paranoid schizophrenia when I was twelve years old. It's a disorder that affects how a person thinks, feels, and acts. Dad, Rachel, and I were told that there are many types of schizophrenia and a lot of misinformation about the disorder. While often confused with multiple personality disorder in popular culture, it is completely unrelated to this condition. It is not caused by childhood trauma or bad parenting, and those with schizophrenia rarely pose a threat to others. Instead, the way schizophrenia presents in an individual can run the gamut from symptoms like an inability to tell the difference between the real and the imagined to becoming withdrawn or unable to respond appropriately in certain social situations.

The truth is no one knows for certain what causes schizophrenia. The good thing was that Mom was stable at the moment. And I was grateful for that.

After Bobby and I checked out of the hotel, we grabbed coffees and sandwiches at Starbucks and then headed to Ocean Shores, where Mom had been living in a small summer cabin. It was a two-and-a-half-hour drive from Seattle to Aberdeen, where Mom had worked, and then another half hour to Ocean Shores.

Bobby and I didn't say much during the drive. We simply enjoyed the scenery and the comfort of knowing that Mom had a new place to live.

As we approached Aberdeen, I saw that it was a town filled with quaint cottages and boutiques. Probably the most famous thing about Aberdeen is that it's the hometown of Nirvana members Kurt Cobain and Krist Novoselic. In fact, a welcoming sign for visitors to Aberdeen proclaims "Come as You Are": a tribute to the band.

What I remembered most about Kurt Cobain, though, was that I had sobbed when he died. I loved Nirvana's music. And I loved Kurt Cobain. "Come as You Are" would continue playing in my mind over and over even after his death, as if it could save me from the nightmare I was living.

"Did you know that at the turn of the twentieth century Aberdeen was a notorious Western outpost?" asked Bobby.

"Really?" I knew Bobby was just trying to make conversation.

"I googled it," he said. "It was a lawless place full of whorehouses and gambling dens. In the early 1900s, it was known as the 'Hellhole of the Pacific' for its high murder rate."

"I never knew that. But it's fitting." For me, Aberdeen was the place where my mother had worked when she suffered a stroke. That nickname rang true.

CHAPTER SIX

Burnt Candles

Look into the crystal ball.
I can see my life begin to fall
to the ground.
Look around me
I can see the hateful smiles
at home.
I feel all closed up
at home.

—Karena, age twelve

Dreary.

That's how it felt when Bobby and I wound our way to Ocean Shores. Mom had found this place when she first arrived in Washington after she obtained a social worker job. When she showed me pictures, I thought it looked charming. But in person, it seemed abandoned and timeworn, particularly in the dead of winter. There was something melancholy about the area. It was a seafaring community that had long ago lost its seamen and fishing boats and felt a bit out of touch with the rest of the world. As if life had passed it by and it had remained a spectral image of itself, like one of those ghost towns.

As we drove to the entrance of the tourist area where Mom lived, a sea-washed blue sign hung at the entrance: "Welcome to Ocean Shores." A low-lying fog spread over the ground and shrubs as if hiding their true colors.

It was February, and as with most days in the Pacific Northwest winter, it was rainy and gray. We drove down a paved road and found her cabin at the end, nestled in between trees. Leaves scattered across the driveway, and tall grass blew in the wind.

My heart caught in my throat as we approached. A small brown-framed wooden house with a front porch, it also looked like a place that time had forgotten. A place where people had given up on their dreams or where a formerly homeless person might take refuge. Where, at nighttime, the trees would shake with ominous whispers.

It could have been cute if there had been any signs of life surrounding it. If there had been flowers, or a couple of chairs on the deck, or a grill on the porch. If it looked like a family visited on vacation during the summers. *Anything.* But this was a place where Mom had hidden away from most of the world.

A small blue car sat in the driveway, looking as lonely as the cabin.

Mom had lived here for a year and a half after staying with Bobby and me in California. I often wondered if she blamed me for her predicament in Washington. After all, she had wanted to stay with us and work for my company, but I wouldn't let her.

I thought back to that time and remembered that I hadn't seen her for three or four years before she just showed up at our door in Manhattan Beach. Bobby and I hadn't been living together very long, and we were both taken aback when she arrived out of the blue. I was happy to see Mom, though, and I set her up in our spare bedroom for her "visit."

Unfortunately, Mom's behavior was strange, and she'd stayed holed up in her bedroom for hours without talking to us. We also noticed that she wasn't doing well physically. Whenever we were out walking to a restaurant or somewhere else, she'd have to stop every few feet to rest on a curb.

I begged Mom to see a doctor. I wasn't aware at the time that she had a bleeding disorder and was hiding it from me. She blamed bottled water and tried to convince us that we were all being poisoned. Only later did I understand why she was so weak.

"They're putting poison in bottled water to kill people," she said. She warned us about documents reporting a grand conspiracy to kill everyone through bottled water, and specifically through the type we bought. We were careful to not bring that water into the house while she was there.

"Mom, it's OK. We're not being poisoned. We're fine, I promise you," I repeatedly told her. Bobby and I just looked at each other. He was as worried as I was. We both knew she was not well.

One night, trying to be positive, I said, "Mom, you've been doing very well. We're all going to be fine."

She retreated to her bedroom and slammed the door. During the rest of her visit, Mom became more withdrawn, suspicious, and cold. Of course, that should have been a warning sign that she was becoming unhinged.

"It's only temporary," I later told Bobby when he asked how long she'd be with us.

Bobby was on edge. So was I. I cooked all the meals and made sure they were nutritious. I bought Mom special vitamins and organic food and did everything I could to make her comfortable. But at night, discouraged with the reality of the situation, I'd retreat to my bedroom and sob.

The truth was that I wanted my mother back—the one I had when I was five years old, before all her symptoms started to appear. I wanted a mother now with whom I could talk about mutual interests in art, fitness, and creativity. I wanted us to go to the salon and have our hair cut and styled and our nails manicured. I wanted us to go shopping and pick out cute clothes. If only we could have had lunch at a charming bistro and drink wine and talk about silly, girlie stuff. If only she could have been more of a mom.

When I look back, I believe I wanted Mom to hold me—*the little girl*—and say in a soothing voice, "Karena, I'm here for you, *dear one*, and everything is going to be all right."

It never happened.

One day, as Bobby watched me struggling to make Mom happy, he spoke up, his voice growing louder with each word. "Karena, I know your mom is sick, but she's not doing anything to help herself and she's draining you . . . and we need our home back. We need our lives back."

"I know." My voice sounded small.

"We have to figure something out." He was exasperated. "You're devoting all your time to caregiving."

I didn't respond. I didn't mean to do it purposefully, but I found myself shutting Bobby out when I didn't want to *go deep*. It was just too painful.

"Karena, c'mon, please, let's talk about this . . . about what we're going to do . . . about your mom . . . and . . . everything."

"Look, I feel like shit about all of this," I said. "But she's my mom, and I don't want to talk about this right now. I'll take care of it."

Truth was, I simply couldn't handle it. I loved Bobby and I loved Mom. But I just couldn't talk about it or even think about the way I could reconcile the two.

That night in bed, Bobby and I got under the covers and he cradled my body, whispering that everything would be OK and that we would work things out. Finally, listening to his soft, rhythmic breathing, I relaxed and fell asleep in his arms.

The next day, I was prepared to ask Mom to leave, but before I could, she decided she would leave on her own. She had a thirteen-year-old dog, Cedar, who was a pit bull–Lab mix. He had been her travel companion for a long time. I didn't particularly like him because he would chase my cats, but he was good to Mom, and I felt better that he'd be with her.

I tried to convince her to go see a doctor before leaving because I knew her mental illness was taking over again.

"I don't have health insurance," she said, "and I want to wait until I get a job."

"OK," I told her. "But promise me you'll go see a doctor as soon as you get health insurance."

Mom nodded.

"And just where are you going?" I asked.

"Hood River, Oregon," she said. "I have a friend there. I've been researching the area online for a while. I've read it's beautiful. I'll be surrounded by nature, and the air is nice. I should be able to find a job."

Mom had a habit of running away. She always thought that somewhere else would bring her peace. That she could escape herself.

"That's wonderful, Mom. Oregon is a great state."

Bobby and I were both overjoyed to hear that she had a friend in Oregon. I breathed a sigh of relief.

On the day she left, I hugged her goodbye and told her to let me know where she was living when she arrived. Mom and Cedar got in her car. As she pulled out of the driveway, I stood there, waving. But she didn't look back.

We rejoiced in having our home back. In having our privacy back. Our lives.

That joy didn't last long.

A couple of weeks later, Mom called. I asked how things were, and she said, "I can't find a job here. Things aren't working out, Karena. I need to leave."

"I'm sorry," I said. "Sometimes things work out if you stick with them for a while."

"I've been thinking," she said. "Why don't I come back to your place and work for your company? I could take some fitness classes, get in shape, and be a success story for your company."

I was caught off guard.

Finally, I stammered, "Mom—um—there aren't any job openings, and I don't think that would be a good idea."

"All right, Karena," she said curtly.

Why do I feel so guilty? I thought.

"Don't worry about me. I'll be just fine." Her tone sounded judgmental.

I couldn't let her pull me into her drama. I couldn't let her make me feel any guiltier than I already did.

"Let me know where you go," I said finally.

From what she later told me, she had moved around to different areas before settling in Washington. Mom had money that she had saved when she worked in Florida, but she soon spent all of it. At one point, she ended up in Monterey, California, sleeping in her car at night. Sometimes she would call me and let me know where she was, and I'd deposit money in her bank account for her. Occasionally

I booked a room for her at some affordable motel so she could have a bed and a hot shower.

One night, when she called, I told her that I had booked her a room for two weeks.

"I'd rather sleep in my car, Karena. I've heard there might be bedbugs in motels."

What?

Bedbugs?

I couldn't believe she'd rather sleep in her car, where she would be cold and uncomfortable, than have a nice, warm room in a motel. Sure, small motels weren't the Taj Mahal, but they were safe, warm, and clean. And there were hot showers.

I knew Mom was in a delusional state and there was nothing I could do.

After Monterey, she drove to Colorado and moved into a friend's house. At first, I was relieved that she was actually living with a friend. But after three weeks, she called and said, "Karena, my friend is a Satan worshipper and I have to get out of here."

I was distraught.

What am I going to do? I thought. *Is this a delusion or is there really some reason Mom is unsafe there?*

Mom was distraught too.

"Look, Mom, if you really believe she's a Satan worshipper, then get out of there now. You've mentioned Washington before. Why don't you go there? If you need some money, I'll help you out, but just go."

I didn't want her to come back to California, but I did want her to find a place where she felt happy, safe, and secure. Mom agreed that she'd try Washington. Luckily, she later called to tell me she'd found a job as a social worker in Aberdeen, Washington, and had arranged for an interview.

"That's great, Mom," I said. "Hey, I'll get you a hotel room beforehand so you can be fresh for the interview."

"No, that's not necessary, Karena. I'll just sleep in my car."

"You can't do that," I said. "I'll book you a hotel room for a couple of weeks. That way, you can clean up for the interview, and then if you get the job, you'll have time to find a place to live."

Mom finally agreed to that. I was a bit surprised that she was healthy enough to attend an interview, but I shouldn't have been. She had always found jobs fairly easily in social work. She had good experience and presented herself very well. She could be extremely personable and friendly. People liked her. She got the job and, shortly after moving to Washington, found the cabin in Ocean Shores.

—

I thought all was well until it came time for my wedding in July. Bobby and I had chosen Hawaii as the destination for an intimate wedding with just forty guests, and I worried whether Mom could handle that trip physically or emotionally. In addition, she told me she didn't want to attend if Dad was coming.

Dad and I had a good relationship. We visited each other often, and I wanted him and my stepmother at my wedding. She was a wonderful woman, and we were all good friends. Mom had not seen Dad for almost twenty years. They hadn't seen or spoken to each other since the day she left him permanently. Dad had tried time and again to meet with her over the years to resolve their old issues, but she always refused. She hated him and blamed him for most of her problems.

I asked Mom to meet with Dad in a neutral place so they could get reacquainted before the event. I was worried about what would happen at the wedding otherwise.

But she was adamant. "No, I will not talk to your father, Karena. But I promise I will be on good behavior at the wedding."

"But it's going to be a small wedding," I said. "You have to talk to him."

She pretended to understand, but she still wouldn't meet with him. After giving it some thought, I told her she was no longer invited. Given her schizophrenia, I couldn't trust how Mom might behave. I didn't want the day to be about her.

I knew that it would be a while before I heard from her. And I was right. She didn't talk to me for months, refusing to return my calls or texts. I sent Mom a necklace that commemorated our wedding. When she didn't acknowledge that she received it, I thought she was giving me the silent treatment.

I offered to visit Mom in Washington to celebrate her new job and share wedding stories with her. She didn't call me back because, I assumed, she was still mad at me. I was so upset, I started therapy again. We wouldn't speak again until after the call from Deborah.

—

"What are you thinking?" Bobby asked, interrupting my thoughts as I shuffled toward the cabin. I was often distracted by memories, as if I could somehow rewrite them and make history different.

"Oh, just remembering how Mom got here in the first place," I said.

"If it hadn't been for you, she wouldn't have been able to rent this house or have this stability at all."

"I know. It's just more dismal than I thought it would be." I motioned toward the building.

"Yeah. Depressing," Bobby said. "Kind of grim."

"Let's just go in and clear it out as fast as we can."

"I'm for that." Bobby picked up his pace, hauling the garbage bags and cleaning supplies we had picked up earlier at a local Ace Hardware store nearby.

Both of us were accustomed to the brilliant sunshine and cloudless skies in California. It made this mist-shrouded area look even darker and more ominous by contrast.

When we stepped through Mom's front door, I looked around at the sparse furnishings. There wasn't much there.

"Look, your mom must have liked burning candles." Bobby pointed to the kitchen countertop where there were about fifty burnt candles piled in a box.

"Maybe the electricity was turned off," I said. "Or maybe there were a lot of storms and that's why the electricity was off."

"Or maybe she used them for meditating," Bobby said. "Or warding off evil spirits." He gave me a look. He knew of Mom's obsessions with conspiracy theories and evil entities.

"Maybe."

The past rushed at me as I faced the current situation. My throat tightened. I almost couldn't breathe.

Perhaps the burnt candles were symbolic of her burning through her life. Did she think burning them would keep her safe from evil?

Did she burn one candle per day? One per week? Or several at once? Did she sit and gaze into the light, trying to perform magic spells? Did she pray with the candles?

What were they used for?

The cabin was small, and I headed for the bedroom. There was an old, dilapidated suitcase in the middle of the floor, and not much else. I packed up all of Mom's clothes that hung in her closet. They fit in that one suitcase. I made a note on my mental list to go shopping for her and buy her some new clothes and shoes. I stripped the sheets and sleeping bag from her bed. They smelled musty and dirty.

I went back out to the living room and sat down on the sofa. It was a very emotional moment for me. I realized the walls of this cabin had contained a life that was dysfunctional and sick. Between these walls, there was nothing. It was empty.

I compared my life with Mom's. I saw her life as lonely and depressing. I, on the other hand, lived a happy, fulfilling, loving life. Mom had been running away from herself for her entire life. As if she was afraid to stop and face herself. She had gone through tragedies and illnesses. It was so sad. Mom's life was empty, and the emptiness in that cabin was a reflection of her. That cabin had known only the delusions of my mother. It was a place that mirrored the neglected pieces of a soul that had lived in utter despair.

In the kitchen, Bobby opened the fridge and found old takeout and emptied water bottles filled with blood. We guessed she'd been vomiting blood into the bottles.

Trash, consisting of empty vodka bottles, take-out boxes, and more blood-filled water bottles, was piled high in the garbage can in the kitchen corner. The rest of the cabin was practically empty except for a few basic pieces of old furniture. A bed, a kitchen table, an uncomfortable sofa, and a couple of chairs.

On the table were a few items that must have been important to her, laid out in a row, as if she had been taking inventory. There were some prayer cards, an empty flower vase, some incense, and a greeting card from me that she had saved from a past Mother's Day. On the edge of the table was the necklace I had made especially for her with the coordinates of my wedding carved in a gold plate with three small diamonds. Mom eventually told me she never received the necklace in the mail, even though I had checked the FedEx tracking number and knew that she had signed for it. It hurt my feelings to see it lying there.

Ready to burst into tears, I took the necklace, rubbed my fingers lovingly over the coordinates, and put it into my purse to take home.

Move on, I told myself. *Don't get distracted by painful memories.*

There were a few paint samples on the table along with a paint swatch of lavender, which was her favorite color. Apparently, Mom had intended to paint the place.

We packed up her computer and a few other personal items that were in the bedroom. We put her stuff into the garbage bags, then started to clean the entire place with bleach.

Suddenly, I realized I had to get out of there.

I couldn't breathe.

"I'm going to her car and see what's in there," I told Bobby.

"You OK, Karena?" he asked. "You look pale."

"I just need some air."

Outside, I started going through her car. I found Mom's journal and a wedding card that she had never sent me. They were piled among more empty food boxes and an almost-empty can of Pringles. In the glove box was a Slim Jim. Her diet had consisted of frozen dinners, takeout, and junk food. And to think, this was a mother who used to be obsessed with healthy food and exercising when I was a little girl. A mother who cooked tofu and made me and Rachel drink SlimFast so we would stay thin.

When I picked up Mom's journal—a spiral notebook—I opened it for just a tiny glimpse. One line hit me hard:

Unfortunately, life has not been a beautiful journey and it has been riddled with much pain and confusion.

I always felt responsible for my mom's life. As if I could have done more to make her happy. To make her more comfortable. I tended to blame myself for so many of Mom's issues, which I knew *intellectually* was not right. But I have always been one who listened more to my heart than my mind.

I looked at the back of Mom's journal and found a shopping list. She had written to-do lists all her life. I've always been the same way, creating lists for everything in my life as a way to organize my days.

- *Sunday*
- *Go to drugstore*
- *Silver jewelry polish*
- *Toilet paper*
- *Chicken pot pie*
- *Buy beef jerky*
- *Buy potato chips*
- *Buy more candles*

Mom always loved her silver jewelry. So that made sense. But the rest of the list seemed to me like something a high school or college student would have written.

I had to close Mom's journal or I would start sobbing right there. I got out of her car and put the journal and her other personal items in our rental car.

I looked up and saw Bobby approaching.

"Are you ready to go?" I asked.

"I think we have everything cleaned out. Yes, we can go."

"That's good," I said. "I don't think I can take much more of this."

"I know. It really is a dismal place, and, well . . . time to get out of here."

"Tomorrow, we can coordinate getting Mom out of the hospital and on a plane to California to her new home."

"That'll be good."

Bobby and I headed to a bed-and-breakfast where we had reserved a room. On the way, we were awestruck by the beautiful sunset off in the distance. We veered off the main highway, parked the car, jumped out, and ran a quarter of a mile down a grassy path to the seashore to watch the sun.

I thought the sunset would help heal me in part, and I was right. Something beautiful in this dreary place. I wanted to stop at the beach after leaving the cabin to memorialize this area as an official place of mourning an end. I wanted to leave the past behind and, in turn, hope for a resurrection of sorts, for Mom to have a new life.

CHAPTER SEVEN

Wild Sorrow

sit in silence
hide my violence
scream inside
you try to hide

—Karena, age twelve

Beautiful.

Not this situation. Not this heartache. But this sunset. Colors fading from salmon to crimson. Ribbons of periwinkle seeping into the horizon. The stunning sunset lured us off the highway and down a side road that led to the ocean.

"Karena, be careful," Bobby called after me as I ran on slippery rocks and driftwood toward the water.

I ignored him. I let go with wild abandon and breathed in the sunset. I needed to be with nature for a little while and escape. I needed to shake off the sorrow that would consume me if I wasn't careful.

Advertising for this beach was splashed on a sign at the beginning of the road. It read: "Great for clamming and kite-flying!" But I saw no sign of life here except for nature in its natural state. No clamming. No kite-flying. Instead, it was quiet. And that's what I needed. The quiet.

The air smelled of salt and fish, which reminded me of ancient mariners. Waves rolled forward, dark and gritty, as though a great knife had been plunged deep into the sea's murky heart. And then, as if acknowledging my broken soul, the waves began to whisper sounds of solace. They slowed to a gentle tumble toward the shore, scattering splintered wood and debris—a mixture of gray and charred black—while I found my footing and then steadied myself on an old tree trunk.

Seashores are often too loud—the waves too powerful, too deafening—to hear my own bruised and bleeding thoughts when I'm upset, so I used to scream at the sea when I was heartbroken or anxious or scared. But now . . . *nothing.* My voice was gone. I was wavering between suffocating silence and holy admiration for the most beautiful sunset I'd ever seen.

I couldn't help it. Emotions washed over me along with gritty, painful memories. I could not stop crying. I watched the sunset from my perch and felt the tears trickle down my cheeks and into my mouth, wet and salty, as the wind whipped my long hair across my face. I cried until my tears became those of the angels. For wasted time. For lost things. For fleeting moments of love that long ago became too frail, too fragile, too crumbly to hold on to forever. For family memories that were imagined but never created. For goodbyes to a life that could have been. For lost souls and a mother who wasn't really there. For things that could not be mended no matter how hard I tried.

I stood tall against the wind, shoulders back, heart and soul surrendering as the sun drifted rose colored into the sea, casting a soft pale glow over the debris of washed-up wood, splintered and strewn across the seagrass. I gazed out over the sea through blurry eyes, becoming lost in the rhythmic percussion of waves on the shore. I felt the acute pain of wild sorrow as I acknowledged untended wounds, the scars deep in my bones. I wasn't sure I would ever be completely healed. Or whole. I told myself that it's a continuing process. I told myself that it's OK. I'll get better each day. I know I will.

I reminded myself: *Mom is not dead; she is still here.* But in so many ways, she died a long time ago. Death is always standing close by. A pale skeletal figure shrouded in a long black coat, fiery-red eyes of hell, burning holes through his hood, wielding a scythe in his hand, vigilantly waiting.

I shivered, sucking in the cold. The sea air bit into me like ice. I wrapped my arms tighter around my body. For a second, the world flickered into darkness. As if this wild sorrow were trying to consume me. I knew it was. But I wouldn't let it.

Yes, things were scary. Frustrating. Life-changing.

But the sunset—this was a thing of beauty, despite the fractured, loud seashore. This was a place where heaven and earth met, and in a transcendent moment, it had become part of an experience of awe and respect for what we call "life." And the moments to come were yet to be revealed. I could turn those moments into transcendence too.

My mother had broken my heart a thousand times, but little by little, she opened me to a wider sense of identity. Because of her, I became capable of seeing through the illusions of people in a world with mental disorders. I could read between the lines and knew the difference between someone who abandons you or lashes out at you because of their own insecurity and fear and someone who acts mean because they are an unkind person. A broken heart had taught me how to thrive *in spite of* grief.

It was a broken heart that could let slip into its core the delight of shimmering paints on a canvas, the wonder of Mozart, and the sheer beauty of sunlight dappling through leaves. It was a broken heart that understood how life-affirming messages of hope and love could be revealed in a glorious sunset on a deserted coastal road.

I was aware that Bobby was taking photos of me. He didn't know how to "fix" my heartache. He wasn't sure what to say, and I didn't know how to help him console me. After all, he grew up in a supportive family in Long Island, New York, where love was taken for granted. Where two parents came together in body, heart, and mind for their children's best interests. *Where he was loved.* And it was never a question. We didn't have the same life challenges. The hardships made me defiant and gave me a stronger purpose. And yet, I knew the pain and difficulties in my life affected Bobby too.

"C'mon, Karena, we need to go." His voice was soft and gentle; he knew if it was too loud, too insistent, I might break. And I knew that if I glanced at him, I would see his strong, broad shoulders, sun-kissed blond hair, and the kindest pale-blue-green eyes, desperately wanting to take the pain away from me. But this was mine. This pain was singular, and in many ways, I wanted to protect him from it. But we shared everything; it had been this way ever since we met.

The sun was sinking faster now, and the whole sky turned crimson. The waves below me seemed quieter, and suddenly I understood more clearly why I had to stop and watch this transcendent sunset by the ocean.

When you get stung in life, go to the Sea of Renewal, where, through alchemy, the waters will heal you, the sea whispered to me. The sea had always been a place of renewal for me.

Yes! I responded quietly to myself. *That's it!* Yes, I would transform despair into regeneration and renew my life for the better. I would help my mom heal and start over too. I would take this opportunity to give Mom life, just as she gave me mine. We would truly get to know each other and build a loving relationship. This was another chance for me. And it was another chance for Mom. I would use this time, this energy, to help create self-empowerment for us both.

Thank you, I said inwardly to the Sea of Renewal. The ocean had given me what I needed.

Full of renewed hope, I smiled faintly, wiping the tears from my eyes, and turned from the sea, hurrying back to where Bobby was waiting.

—

Standing on that seashore at sunset, I found new strength. I heard the call of the Sea of Renewal and was given the courage to move onward.

That night, after we grilled salmon steaks on our little patio at the bed-and-breakfast, I curled up in front of a fire and read more of my mother's journal. I wouldn't normally do something like this, but I wanted to understand the mental state she was in. I wanted to know what I was dealing with.

And I sobbed. For her loneliness. Her despair. Her deep depression. Bobby cuddled me.

"I feel like I've let her down somehow. How could I have allowed her to get to this state?"

"Karena, it's OK to not take care of everyone and everything," he said. "This isn't your fault. Her happiness is not your responsibility.

And you can't be expected to take this on all by yourself. You shouldn't have to. You're way too hard on yourself. I'm here, and I will always be here to help you."

But I couldn't help feeling my mom's pain. It hurt deeply to know how much suffering the woman who gave me life was experiencing. I believe that we feel the hurt when those we love are in pain.

As I fell asleep in Bobby's arms, the firelight casting long shadows on the walls, I was reminded that a *renewal* has many things to teach us. It gives us the opportunity for new growth and a better life. But there will still be difficult times as we move forward toward peace, healing, and clarity.

Remember, the firelight seemed to whisper, *the Sea of Renewal means this is a time for change. For rebirth. For resurrection. For a new beginning.*

PART TWO

Genesis of Family

CHAPTER EIGHT

"Ya Tebe Lyublyu"

"Good Soil"
Dedicated to Nick's parents
Song and lyrics by Nick Ivanovich

You were displaced from your home in Ukraine.
You knew you couldn't stay when the
    Communists came.
So you headed down the road that shook under
    your feet.
Remaining steadfast in your journey to be free.

Traveling that dark passage to a camp in West
    Germany
With images of the war haunting your memory.
It was at that time there were two children to
    feed.
What waited your tomorrows was hard to
    conceive.

Like scattered seeds that fell on good soil.
That keep yielding crops in these lives of ours.

Your hope in returning home went up in flames.

Missed loved ones to never see again.
So to America you flew to start a new life.
To live that dream that would not be denied.

Hands to the plow, you never looked back.
With dirt on your hands and your body wracked.
And the legacy you left you will forever endure.
I see it in me and my children for sure.

DNA.

We all come from somewhere. We all have a lineage, the genesis, our beginnings.

I was born with DNA that was forged with strength and courage long ago.

I have been fortunate. My hardships in life have been nothing compared to what my grandparents experienced. If it had not been for their courage, their strength, their love for family, I would not be here today. And my family would not be here. I am certain about that.

I remember talking to Bobby about the beginnings of my family when he asked me where I got my passion, my courage. "I was born with it. I got it from my grandparents. And those before them."

My babushka would smother us with kisses.

Babushka would wrap us in her arms so tightly, I could smell flour and cinnamon and blueberries on her apron and feel the pounding of her heart. I knew my grandmother loved me, and I loved her fiercely in return.

Babushka loved to cook for us, and that included everything from *varenyky*, a Ukrainian dumpling filled with blueberries; to *holubtsi*; to kielbasa; to *paska*, a bread decorated with braids. During holidays, she would stand in the kitchen and prepare huge meals of fried chicken and borscht and noodles. We children—Sasha, the nickname we gave Rachel (and she nicknamed me Sissy), my cousins, and I—would sit at a separate table in a side room, listening as the adults laughed and talked and drank wine at the main dining table in the kitchen. I always wanted to be a part of their conversation and learn their secrets.

The truth is, it's a wonder these warm memories ever happened, that my sister and I were born at all. If my father's parents had been killed in Ukraine—as planned by the Nazis—then I would not even be a memory. My mother and father would not have met, and Rachel and other relatives wouldn't exist. There would be no chain connecting mother to daughter, sister to sister, or father to daughter. We would have all been lost to each other, and these family memories would never be.

We all have beginnings, and in those humble beginnings are our memories. For me, the memories of my Ukrainian grandparents are some of the best. Even now, I smile with a full heart when I think of them.

In one memory, when I must have been only four years old, I am pulling cucumbers from the vines that scrambled along the ground in Babushka's huge vegetable garden at my grandparents' home in Peru, Indiana. Sometimes the cucumber plants would clamber up trellises and be easy to reach, but I mostly recall the ones on the ground. I remember the spiky points on the dark-green skins that sometimes pricked my fingers. I remember the cucumbers' clean, fresh smell, similar to that of a watermelon. I remember big toads croaking throaty "ribbit" sounds as they leaped away from my hands near the cucumber vines. Sometimes slimy slugs clung to the vines, creating an obstacle for me to reach the cucumbers.

I remember putting the cucumbers in a wicker basket that was almost bigger than I was and carrying it back to Babushka, where she would wash and slice them into thin wafer-like pieces and then let them marinate in vinegar and salt.

Not far from the garden, I would walk through dew-covered vines in Babushka's vineyard and steal big purple grapes, even though I knew they were scheduled to be harvested soon for wine. Sasha would tell me that I wasn't supposed to eat the grapes. Sometimes I could be bossy, even at four years old, according to Sasha, and I'd put my hands on my hips, stomp my feet, and shout, "You can't tell me what to do!"

I didn't stay angry with her for long, though. I loved my Sasha, and as she watched me stuff the grapes into my mouth, juice dribbling down my chin, she would giggle and join in. If we heard any adults approaching, we'd run and hide between the grape arbors, taking cover under a shady canopy of beautiful foliage.

These were idyllic times when Mom and Dad were still the perfect parents. When they were still in love, and we were still the perfect family.

My father's parents, Babushka and my grandfather, whom we called Geed (pronounced with a soft *G*, as in George), lived through the great Soviet famine in Ukraine in the 1930s and were nearly executed by Nazi soldiers who invaded the country in 1941. My grandparents barely escaped being killed. Life was difficult for all the Soviet citizens in the 1940s. Consumer goods were scarce, and there was extensive hunger everywhere. Little pay and crowded housing conditions were the norm.

"In our rural village," Babushka once reminisced, "we women wore long, billowing peasant dresses and scarves on our heads. We had to fill buckets with water from wells and streams, and position them on the ends of long poles, then hoist them on our shoulders and walk miles and miles across fields and forests to our homes. Our homes were huts, generally not much more than one-room buildings, and we heated them and lit the rooms at night with big stone fireplaces and oil lamps. To cook, we built fires in brick ovens and stone fireplaces."

"It sounds hard," Sasha said, her eyes wide with sympathy.

"Yes, my dear, life was hard and simple, but there was always love."

That was the thread that held these peasant families together. Likewise, that thread—fragile as it seems sometimes—still holds my family together.

After the Nazi invasion, Babushka's family lived in the woods in makeshift tents. While she was peeling carrots, she recounted all sorts of tales from the old country, and Sasha and I sat around the kitchen table, wide-eyed. "We didn't have much more than the clothes on our backs, and I was pregnant with your *bat'ko*—your papa—and didn't get much to eat. We'd roam the forests for wild berries, and your Geed and the other men would hunt and kill rabbits and squirrels for us to make stew."

Sasha and I could not imagine anyone living in the woods filled with bears and all kinds of wild animals. How did they survive? We had always known that our grandparents were exotic people in many ways, with their thick accents, their ethnic folk songs, and the unusual

clothes that they sometimes wore. And we knew they were hard workers. *But to live in the woods?*

"Why didn't you stay at your home?" Sasha asked.

"Soldiers came to our village and ran us out of our homes."

Babushka described how millions of Ukrainians, including Geed
and herself, were sent to a refugee camp. She also told us how they had
to do hard work there in constant fear of being killed by the Nazis for
no reason at all.

I asked if she was ever afraid they were going to be killed. It was
hard for me at that young age to understand the inhumane way people
sometimes treated others. I knew nothing about the Nazis at that age,
and these stories made me terribly sad.

Babushka nodded. "One time, the Nazis lined up some men in a
ditch along with your grandpapa and started shooting them. Killing
them one by one." Babushka's eyes glazed with tears. I started shaking.

Sasha and I both looked at her with horror. We were just little girls
and had not experienced anything like this.

"I pleaded with them to not kill your grandpapa. Finally, one of
the soldiers took pity on us and spared his life." She took the edge of
her apron and wiped her eyes, not wanting me and Sasha to see her
grief.

I later learned that they were displaced persons—a term for millions of people worldwide, many of whom had been put into camps for
forced labor during World War II, as well as surviving Jews. There was
no recognized Ukrainian state at the end of World War II, and from
1949 to 1952, thousands of Ukrainian immigrants were authorized to
enter the United States as displaced persons.

Fortunately, my grandparents were eligible. Babushka was pregnant with my father when she and Geed and their two little daughters,
Mary and Helen, along with Geed's brother, immigrated to the United
States. A church in Peru, Indiana, sponsored some of the Ukrainian
refugees, and that's where my grandparents and their family settled. And where my father was born. Geed worked in a factory at the
Chrysler plant in Peru, and Babushka was a homemaker. They created
a good, stable, and loving home for their family.

Many years later, just before I started kindergarten, my parents
moved us from Peru to Indianapolis so my father could get a better

job. After we moved, we only saw my grandparents a couple of times a year, mostly during the holidays.

I was in the second grade when Geed died at the age of sixty-five. Rachel and I cried. Our hearts were broken. I still have a vivid memory of my father sitting on the love seat in the living room of our home in Indianapolis after the funeral. His shoulders were hunched over and shaking. It was the first time anyone we loved had died, and it had a lasting effect on both Rachel and me. It was also the first time I ever saw my father cry.

Babushka lived another twenty years after my grandpa passed away. She never loved another man. She got dementia later in life and died when she was eighty-three years old.

I still miss them every single day.

When I think of the hardships they survived to get to America, I am humbled and grateful. And when I think about the Nazis killing people at random in the refugee camps, I am especially grateful they spared my grandparents, which was a miracle. A beautiful miracle.

Everything I've ever set out to do, I've done with a quiet ferocity and passion that drives me forward. I am not afraid to take risks, and that has propelled me further than I would have ever dreamed. It is the same with love, although through my teens, I nearly forgot that love could heal me. It is because of my grandparents' courage and strength, their DNA, that I am learning how to become stronger in my life. For that, I am forever grateful.

"*Ya tebe lyublyu*, Geed and Babushka." It was one of the only Ukrainian phrases that I can remember from what Babushka taught me: "I love you."

CHAPTER NINE

Descent into Darkness

Demons watch, evil mind
Voices of darkness seem unkind
Drips a tear for Mother's love
Sits in corner, wonders of . . .
(Who can she love?)

Burn a candle, pure as white
Sit real still, straight and tight
Dripping blood, no more stress
Dance around in black dress . . .
(Do you see the demons by your side?)

—Karena, age twelve

Madness.

My mother's descent into darkness was born from a legacy of madness that existed long before we were aware of what was happening. The seeds of her madness began with her parents, who were very different from my father's. Mom's parents didn't escape from the Nazis in a war-torn country. They didn't struggle to survive by living in the woods, roasting rabbits and squirrels. No, they were not refugees who were daily threatened with death by the Nazis. But Mom and her family had their own kind of hardship, which turned out to be just as deadly.

If anyone had looked at my mother's family behind closed doors during the time she was growing up in the 1950s and '60s, it would have been obvious that they lived in their own emotionally war-torn world long before Mom married my father.

And so, I was born with not only the DNA forged with the strength and courage from my Ukrainian grandparents but also the DNA from my mother's family that perpetuated brilliance and derangement. From that lineage, some might assume that I was destined to follow in the footsteps of the mentally ill, like my mother and others in her family, and for a while, I thought that would come to be true. I lived the wildest, most rebellious life I could, beginning at eleven years old and continuing into my teens and early twenties.

Little by little, I learned that we are all in charge of our destiny, and I was determined to not follow in the footsteps of my mother's family. I would not become a forgotten footnote in the annals of time due to the effects of a family with mental illness. No, I would not—*will not*—let that be the master of my destiny.

As an adult, I have continually examined what happened when I was a child and have tried to learn valuable lessons from memories of my experiences. I won't let the pain of those memories and experiences kill the heart in me, although they almost did . . . for a while.

As a young girl, I didn't know much about Mom's family. Only that she grew up in a middle-class neighborhood in Muncie, Indiana, in the 1960s, and that she had one brother and a sister and varied pets throughout her childhood. Her parents were of Irish and German descent, raised in families that had lived in the US for many generations.

From what Mom has said, she and her siblings were all smart children who made good grades and enjoyed the normal, everyday things that children in the '60s experienced. Table tennis. Church cakewalks. Piano lessons. Fall festivals at school. Riding bikes. Picnic lunches of peanut-butter-and-jelly sandwiches. They were the *Leave It to Beaver* type of family that looked perfect when they sat together in the church pews on Sundays: Mom and her sister, Carol, wearing dresses, hats, and patent-leather shoes. A Norman Rockwell painting.

But, according to Mom, they were anything but perfect. Strange, scary events happened in the dark, at night, behind closed doors. Things started unraveling when her father became obsessed with the occult. He had a violent temper that got worse when he drank liquor, and he drank nightly. He cursed at them, telling them that God would send them to hell. He threw dishes as the family sat at the dinner table, the plates shattering on the floor as they ducked to dodge his anger. He whipped the girls with tree branches until they had bleeding welts on their legs. He screamed at them, and then he beat them if they talked back to him.

Mom's mother was a quiet, nondescript figure in the background who didn't appear to have much influence over her demented husband or the household. The type of mother in the 1950s and '60s who let the husband run the roost, never questioning him or demanding him to be anything other than narcissistic and controlling. If beating was part of that scenario, then so be it.

Professionally, Grampa was a high achiever in his career and was vice president of a family business. He was also a brilliant scientist, an inventor who was included in the *Who's Who* book twice for his accomplishments. But he was also delusional, a violent tyrant and alcoholic who had been diagnosed with a psychotic disorder and schizophrenia.

I remember Grammy as being kind and sweet to me and Rachel. She was creative too, and taught me and Rachel how to knit and crochet hats and scarves. Grammy let me and Rachel play dress-up whenever we visited, and it was one of our favorite things to do. We would dress in her chunky high heels, clothes, and hats from the 1950s and help her bake cookies in the kitchen. We knew that Babushka and Geed had survived the horrors of the Nazis and a world war; we didn't know that Grammy had survived her own terror living with Grampa and his violence. While Babushka and Geed escaped to the United States, Grammy was not to escape her specific type of horror in middle-class 1950s USA until Grampa died.

When I asked Mom how Grammy reacted to Grampa's violent temper and drinking, she shrugged. "Mom was quiet about it. Married women in the 1950s were supposed to be good wives and let the men be in charge of the families. The men would beat them if they defied them. So she mostly didn't say anything when he beat us. I imagine many homes were like ours. The wife quietly sat by and watched her husband do anything he wanted, whether it was drinking or beating the children or her.".

When Mom was a teenager, Grampa descended into his own madness, eventually dying by suicide after getting drunk and driving his car into a tree.

It was shocking to the whole neighborhood and to my mom, but I'm not sure she grieved his death. She might have been happy about it. After all, once he died, they no longer had to endure the beatings or rantings of a depraved madman.

Everything takes its toll, eventually, though. I've understood as an adult that Mom experienced her own heartbreaks because of her dysfunctional childhood. Insecurity and paranoia were seeded in my mother's psyche early on.

So when my father met my mother in the 1970s, she was already carrying her own neuroses with her. They were embedded in her DNA, along with mental illness.

Dad understood Mom better than most because of his education and training in psychology and work as a psychotherapist. We often talked about it, especially when he would later visit me in California.

—

I had just picked Dad up at the airport in LA and was driving him to my house for a visit. The good memories of my childhood were sparse, and although his perspective was somewhat different from mine, I needed his input on what had happened in our lives. I needed to know more about this ache in my heart that hadn't healed.

"There were a number of years that things seemed like they were going OK for us," he told me. "Your mom and I were raising you and Rachel, my work as a therapist was thriving, I was enjoying my freelance career as a singer-songwriter, and life was good."

"I know," I said. "I remember some good times too. Mom encouraged me and Rachel to do art, and we both loved that. She had her good moments. Did you know right away when you met Mom that she might have some mental health problems?"

"Actually, it wasn't until we'd been married for about ten years that I really started to notice strange things about her behavior," Dad said.

"I already knew that Linda had a very troubled adolescence. Her father's delusions were really scary. When we started dating, she shared those things with me and confided how discouraged she was about relationships, in general. Our own relationship was rocky in the beginning. I was young, in my early twenties, and had not had that much experience with women. But your mom . . . well, she had one of the most beautiful faces I had ever seen. Deep-blue eyes and the most gorgeous smile. And, at times, she could be so creative and inventive. She intrigued me, I have to say."

"Weren't you in graduate school, studying psychology at the time?" I asked. We were at a standstill on the 405 freeway. Bumper to bumper. It was going to be a long drive.

"Yeah, I had taken a course in multiple personalities as part of my psychology curriculum. Linda agreed to do a test for me for my class, and I remember that when the professor looked at the profile of her test, he told me that this person harbored an extremely high level of confusion and paranoia. Even though she didn't seem to be experiencing an active delusional process at the moment, she definitely exhibited a confused state and emotional instability."

"In other words, you were warned," I said, glancing sideways at my father. He had been through his own hell with Mom.

"Uh-huh, I guess so," said Dad. "It scared me a little. I knew how serious these patterns were. And Linda was compulsive about a number of things too. She was a smoker, drank a lot, and was quite promiscuous . . . right out of the hippie era, but I dabbled in that as well, like so many people of my generation, so I understood. We worked through some of our issues, and she seemed OK. She even said that I had a stabilizing effect on her. We broke up once in the early part of our relationship but got back together six months later and then got married in 1977. And then along came Rachel and you. Two beautiful daughters, and for a while, Linda seemed to thrive on being a mother. I thought that you and Rachel would keep her grounded, you know. Like I said, life was really good . . . for a while."

As we drove along the 405 freeway that night, reflecting on the past, my father and I both became quiet. Each of us was lost in private thoughts about what might have been. What might have been if the madness had not descended.

As a child, I thought what had happened to my family was the work of literal demons. And I still wondered how long the demons had watched our family—my generation and the many generations that preceded me—before they found an opening, a portal to descend upon us. Trying their best to devour us. Not caring about the blood in their wake.

Did the demons take joy in each victory? Did they invade every family in some way through the DNA?

There was a full moon in the sky that night as we drove along. Surely, that moon had memories. Surely, that moon had intimately known members of my family, many who were long gone. Their bones turning to dust. Their ashes scattered across the plains.

Whenever I look up at the full moon, it feels private, as though I have peered through a veil of five thousand worlds. I can imagine for a moment what the sky has hidden from most everyone else. I can see where the winds have blown with a weariness over the land, lulling us all to sleep in a cloud of forgetfulness. I can glimpse the moon folding herself into buttery-soft crescents and lopsided half smiles. When I look up, I can imagine an existence as vast and ancient and immortal as the sky. Just as infinite. Just as unknown. And I remember how my DNA contains courage, strength, valor, brilliance, *and* madness. The DNA of my family.

Knowing this, there lingers a mournfulness in me for the broken chains of family in the passage of time. For the misshapen DNA that allows demons and madness to materialize. I recognize that each of us must navigate our ancestry, the world, and society with all the infinite uniqueness of our family history, personalities, individual talents, and proclivities. We must find our place in the beautiful brokenness that is humanity, the beautiful brokenness in our own DNA, in our own souls, and observe, translate, and change—if needed—in the best way possible what we discover along the way.

Unfortunately, not all of us make it. We don't all survive.

But we do have a choice. And we can try.

CHAPTER TEN

When the Demons Arrive

The demons have taken over my land
Satan's feet are planted in the sand.
We all bow down
as God leaves his crown.
My life begins to blur
into one huge color.
The darkness in my head
has caused me to cry in bed.
I have to assume
that my life will end in doom.

—Karena, age thirteen

Demons.

First, there's the arrival of the demons. They edge their way into your personal space—into your home, your school, your bedroom, your life with your friends and your family—slowly, slyly. The demons bring the madness. And the madness can start with small things. So small you barely notice at first that anything is unusual or strange. It's only when the madness takes control and turns your life upside down with pain and cruelty, with sadness and frustration, that you begin to wonder about your own sanity and if there's any escape.

My father, mother, Rachel, and I lived in a two-story Tudor-style brick house with a red roof and front porch; our home was stylish and comfortable. It had been built in the 1930s and had green-and-yellow stained glass windows in the stairwell and a warm cherrywood fireplace in the living room. The house sat on a street corner, opposite a church, and . . . well, I'm pretty sure it was haunted.

Our street in Indianapolis was a quiet place, especially at night. It was a middle-class neighborhood and far too normal for any kind of monster to live among its pretty, oak-lined streets. But inside that house, the demons had already descended, bringing the madness with them.

It became an ordinary thing to hear Mom and Dad fight, screaming and yelling at each other. I didn't know what was wrong, or if other parents did this, but it scared me.

"You're the Antichrist, a demon," Mom screamed at Dad over and over again one night.

"Linda, what the hell are you talking about?" Dad asked.

"Some of Karena's friends' parents are part of this Antichrist group too." Mom squinted her eyes and flashed a mean look at me. "I know they are. And all of you are part of the New World Order. Your plan is to get rid of everyone else. Me included!" I had no idea what she was talking about.

"That doesn't even make any sense." My dad shook his head. He was busy gathering his guitar and music so he could go play with his band at a local café. I couldn't blame him for wanting to get out of the house. Many times, especially when I was younger, I'd go with him and collect tips in a jar. It was always fun.

"Don't lie to me." Mom paced back and forth in the living room, her hands on her hips.

"I guess I'm going to rise up as the Antichrist. Yeah, right. I'll start a world war and destroy every living thing on the planet. You caught me." Dad shook his head again.

Mom had begun preaching this kind of rhetoric weeks ago.

"Don't act like I'm the fool. The Bible says that the Antichrist will be someone we don't suspect."

"You're reading too much into the Bible."

We hadn't gone to church in a long time.

"I'm getting my news about the New World Order on television," Mom said.

Mom would record hours of news channels on VHS tapes and come up with conspiracies based on what they were talking about. She thought they used code words to send secret messages to members of the New World Order. Of course, I didn't know what she meant when she talked about the New World Order. I didn't know that she thought Dad was the head of an emerging clandestine totalitarian government that would rule the world. That he was part of a group that would orchestrate significant political and financial events to achieve world domination.

But, apparently, Dad knew what it meant, and it scared him.

He tried to divert her attention from the conspiracy theories. "Look, Linda, why don't you come and listen to the band tonight? It would be good for you to get out of the house. The girls are old enough to stay by themselves, or they could come too. Remember how Karena loved listening to us play when she was little—she'd collect the tips for me in a jar?"

Dad threw a look at me. "Wanna come tonight, Karena?"

Before I could say anything, Mom began ranting again. "What? You want me to go and sit and watch you play while all those women flirt with you? That's the only reason you want to play in that goddamn band. It's all the attention you get from the women. I'm on to you."

"That's not true, Linda. You know I love playing music. You knew that when you married me. You used to support my music."

"That's before I knew what a cheat and liar you were."

I crawled inside myself and ran up the stairs to hide in the bedroom I shared with Rachel. I didn't want to hear them scream at each other.

Finally, the front door slammed and the car started. Dad was leaving, and Rachel and I were left alone with our mentally ill mom.

Mom's stability had been steadily faltering, although at that time, as a young preteen, I didn't understand what was happening. I just thought she hated us. No matter what we did, we couldn't please her.

I wish she had been more of a regular mom. A *Brady Bunch* mom. She was a social worker and a talented artist. She even started a greeting card company with Aunt Carol. But ventures like this often didn't last because Mom was too unstable to see anything through to the end.

When Mom and I were alone together, she'd divulge private information to me as if I were her best friend. She'd scream, "Your dad messes around with other women. Did you know that?"

"Mom, don't say that." I wanted to shut my eyes and ears to such a thought.

"Well, he does. Why else do you think he comes home late from work and leaves to play music at night? It's to get away from me and you and Rachel. He goes out at night so he can meet up with other women. The music is just an excuse."

Looking back, I wondered how she could say that to me. Did she expect me to carry the emotional pain of her marriage on my shoulders? I was just a kid!

It was an ugly thought, and I couldn't bear it. I had been a daddy's girl when I was little. When it snowed, we'd build an igloo in the front yard and throw snowballs at each other.

The more Mom complained to me about Dad and shared her delusions with me, the more I slowly turned against him. I was no longer a daddy's girl—but I wasn't exactly a momma's girl either. This is when things started to shift in my life. I started to feel alone and abandoned. I didn't know the truth or whom to trust. I began to question everything.

Things had been good with Mom when I was little. I was a creative child with a big imagination, and I was ambitious. I once opened a restaurant in our basement and served meals to my friends. Mostly peanut-butter sandwiches for a nickel. I created a library and insisted that my friends and family check out the books they wanted to read. They had to pay twenty-five cents a day if they were late in returning them. I also built a Barbie village in our basement and put all my Barbie dolls in homes there. And in the fourth grade, I even opened up a school and taught imaginary students and friends.

At age ten, I asked my parents if I could conduct a yard sale to get rid of all the things we no longer needed. I posted signs around the neighborhood and sat in my front yard all weekend, selling items and serving cookies and lemonade. I made $300 that weekend, which was a fortune! I also earned extra money by walking people's dogs. I became the neighborhood dog walker.

Mom thought that all my business endeavors were ingenious. And I took my stash and bought little presents for everyone—I have always loved buying gifts for others.

Mom set up an easel for herself in the basement and encouraged me and Rachel to paint on a side table she set up for us. We both loved painting. And things went very well until Mom started accusing me and Rachel of stealing her ideas. One day, I walked down into the basement and saw several of Mom's paintings lying against a wall on the floor. Someone had slashed them with a knife, ripping them apart. I knew that Rachel would not do this. Dad did not do this. Seeing those paintings with violent slashes scared me.

And yet Mom was into fitness and health for most of my youth. It was normal for me and Rachel to come home in the afternoon after school to see Mom working out. She would stand there in front of the television set, wearing leotards and leg warmers, with her hair pulled back in a ponytail. Kathy Smith VHS tapes were her favorites. But she also loved Denise Austin, Kathy Ireland, and Jane Fonda fitness videos. I was a fan of those fitness instructors, too, and even turned a nook in my bedroom closet into a shrine with pictures of them from magazines.

I thought it would be so cool to be a fitness instructor, and when I was in first grade, I created a vision board and outlined my dreams. Then I created my own fitness video for a class project. *"Hi, I'm Karena. Welcome to my fat-burning cardio toning workout . . ."* Cue the music . . .

Oftentimes, Rachel and I would hurry upstairs after school, change clothes, and join Mom in the living room to work out to Kathy Smith. Mom liked that. She wanted us to do anything we could to be thin like the girls in the workout videos.

When Rachel and I were small, things at home were Norman Rockwell normal. But as we entered our teens, Mom's moods became erratic and strange, and nothing felt normal anymore. In my mind, everything changed very quickly. Almost overnight.

We had attended a nondenominational Christian church for a while when I was a little girl. It was upbeat with a live band, and I enjoyed it. I talked to God often, telling him about my day, my friends, my family, and my dreams. But little by little, I began to believe that God had abandoned my family and me as my parents fought more often and my mom became increasingly delusional. And then I stopped talking to him. Later, my God would become drugs, cigarettes, alcohol, and boys. When we finally stopped going to church together as a family, Mom said it was because Dad had become the Antichrist and the church was involved.

Mom started doing everything she could to make me hate Dad. To make me believe that he was the reason she was so mad and mean to me and Rachel. And for a while, it worked. My relationship with my father throughout junior and senior high school was rotten. I didn't trust him anymore. I had been brainwashed by Mom.

By the time I was eleven years old, I began to stay away from home after school. I'd go to one of my girlfriend's houses for dinner. Sometimes I called to let my parents know, and sometimes I just didn't call at all and Dad would drive his maroon Mazda around the neighborhood, anxiously looking for me, worried. I didn't care.

As Mom became more delusional, I felt more torn. My foundation had been shattered. Crushed. My psyche felt ripped into a thousand pieces. I couldn't trust Dad anymore because Mom turned me against him. I couldn't trust Mom because she screamed and yelled at me when I talked back to her and then, in the next minute, confided in me like I was an adult.

As for Rachel, she escaped to her own world and mostly kept her frustrations to herself. She was into reading and writing, and that's how she coped. I knew she was hurting too. She ended up doing drugs too but didn't confide in me. Her pain was too deep, too intimate.

I began drinking liquor by the time I was twelve. And not long after, I started smoking cigarettes, alternating between Newport Lights and Camels. I thought I looked cool and sophisticated, like the ads of stylish women in magazines who posed with cigarettes in their fingers while talking to handsome young men.

I was slowly sliding into rebellion. There was nothing I could do to control the situation in my home, so the one thing I could control was the way I behaved outside my home.

One night, when I was eleven, I went over to my friend Rebekah's house to spend the night. Her parents had gone to a party, and we were alone. It was exciting for us because it made us feel like adults. We could do anything we wanted.

"Wanna invite some boys over?" I asked.

"Momma said we couldn't have boys over," she said.

"Oh." I'm sure my face showed my disappointment.

"But I have an idea! Wanna check out my parents' liquor cabinet?" Rebekah asked.

My parents didn't have a liquor cabinet. Mom said that drinking liquor was the devil's work. That it would make you do all kinds of bad things and could turn you into a whore. I couldn't imagine what she was talking about. I knew that Dad drank beer when I was younger. And Mom drank wine, but they'd stopped drinking after I was five, and we never had booze in the house after that.

That night, at Rebekah's, the thought of drinking something forbidden was alluring. Seductive. Empowering.

"C'mon, Karena," Rebekah said. "It's downstairs."

Rebekah's basement had been refurbished into a carpeted den with a sofa, chairs, a television, a small refrigerator, and a liquor cabinet. The whole bottom shelf slid out, so the back could be easily reached. Rebekah and I opened the cabinet slowly. There were numerous bottles of everything including whiskey, vodka, gin, and brandy. We didn't want to break anything.

"Here," Rebekah said, selecting a bottle of peppermint schnapps. "This stuff tastes really good."

"OK. Let's do this." I couldn't wait.

"The best way to drink it is to water it down a little, so it's not so strong," said Rebekah. "Makes it taste better too."

I didn't mind if it was strong, but Rebekah was more sensible—and cautious.

We poured water into tall glasses and then added a tiny bit of peppermint schnapps. "Here, we need some ice," said Rebekah.

We stirred the ice into the glasses and then sipped on our drinks. It tasted good. Like minty water. Not bad at all. And I felt so grown up, just like the women I saw in TV movies. We giggled and swooned, quite sure that we were already drunk. One would have thought that Rebekah and I had drunk a whole bottle of schnapps, when, in reality, we only had a little.

But that night made me more defiant than ever. And for a while, I felt more powerful. I was in charge of my life. I would not let myself become a woman like my mother who complained about the world all the time. I would be whomever I wanted to be.

Things became worse between Mom and Dad, and they began fighting more and more. Rachel and I both often skipped dinners at home because we didn't want to hear my parents fight, and this made Mom very angry because dinners were important to her. And mostly, the dinners were good, but we were never quite sure what we were going to get. For a time, Mom became a vegetarian and ordered us to eat tofu burgers and drink some type of diet meal-replacement drink so we could stay thin. Things derailed. Mom even took me to Chicago once to sign me up with a modeling agency because I was tall and skinny. She had an obsession with controlling us and the food we consumed.

Then, out of the blue, Mom began eating meat again. But by this time, Rachel and I had adopted the vegetarian lifestyle. When Mom started cooking meat for dinner, we refused to eat it because of our vegetarianism. She would throw the meat at us and scream, "Eat this or you'll be sorry you didn't!" Generally, the meat landed on the floor, and Rachel and I were sent to our room without dinner.

When I look back, I can see how Mom's anxiety and instability increased as she became more and more insecure in her and Dad's relationship. How she became more and more obsessive, controlling, and paranoid. She believed she was consumed by sin. And that we were consumed by sin. That we were evil and the devil himself was our leader. She believed that her Bible would save her. That maybe the saints, the apostles Paul or John, would come and rescue her. I believe she was actually waiting for them to walk up to the front door and tell her they were there to save her. She didn't go to church anymore, but she became a religious zealot, and in her mind, Dad was her fiercest enemy.

When Rachel and I went to bed at night, we would hear Mom pacing the floor downstairs, praying to God to save her soul. When she thought the rest of us were asleep, she preached and ranted.

I didn't believe it was God she was talking to. I believed it was those demons. I imagined the demons telling her that she had to pay for her sins. And ours. That she had to escape. That she wasn't safe with Dad or us girls.

I do know one thing to be true: As Mom's delusions became worse, the demons became worse. They were ready to take over. They were ready to devour her.

And if they devoured her, they would certainly devour me too.

CHAPTER ELEVEN

A Walk to the Corner Store

Look into the crystal ball,
I can see my life begin to fall
to the ground . . .
Look around me, I can see the hateful smiles at
    "home."
I feel all closed up at "home."
I wish you would shut up.
I won't sit on your furniture,
I'll just stand here and act mature.
You're so unfair, why don't you care?
Standing in the dark,
drop to my knees,
begging you to forgive me, please.
But that's OK, I'll never forgive you.
What I know, only if you knew
maybe I could run into the night
or just stay through one more fight . . .

—Karena, age thirteen

Hunger.

Not for food, though. Sometimes hunger means you need food, and sometimes it means something much more. For me, it meant much more. I was hungry for love. For acceptance. For a mother.

It was a Friday night in late summer the year I was twelve. The leaves were beginning to turn gold and red, and the nights were chilly. And it should have been an ordinary night. If I had had a crystal ball and could have been warned about what was going to happen, perhaps I could have set into motion a series of events that would have prevented it from happening.

And perhaps not.

Rachel and I were home, getting ready to watch a movie with Mom and Dad. Normal as normal could be. "I'm hungry," I said, remembering that I had skipped lunch.

"What's for dinner?" asked Rachel. We had both perused the refrigerator and kitchen cabinets and couldn't find anything but a couple of carrots and some wilted lettuce.

Dad suggested pizza. "Great idea!" said Rachel. It wasn't often that Mom allowed us to order junk food like pizza. But this was movie night, and Mom was more lenient when we had movies to watch.

After work, Dad had brought home a couple of VHS tapes for us: *Sleepless in Seattle* and *Jurassic Park*. Rachel and I voted to watch *Sleepless in Seattle* first because we wanted to see a romance. I was worried that *Jurassic Park* would give me nightmares.

Mom had been sitting on the sofa, staring out the window, not saying much. She had been quiet and somber all night long, which was unusual. I was grateful, though. As long as she and Dad weren't fighting, I was happy.

"Linda, what do you think about ordering pizza?" Dad asked.

She shrugged. "Sounds OK. Look, Nick, why don't you order Domino's and I'll walk down to the convenience store and buy some sodas for us. You can go ahead and start the movie without me. I'll catch up when I'm back."

Rachel and I debated between a veggie pizza with onions and green peppers or an all-cheese pizza, which we knew would be Mom's choice. She was back on her vegetarian kick again. As for sodas, there were times when she thought they were unhealthy, and other times when she didn't care if we drank them. She was inconsistent.

"It doesn't matter what kind you order," Mom said. She stood up and grabbed her purse and walked out of the house.

Dad ordered Domino's, and we inserted the VHS tape into the player on the shelf under the TV set and started watching *Sleepless in Seattle*.

The delivery driver was timely and brought our pizza in twenty minutes. Dad set the pizza boxes on the coffee table. The delicious aroma of veggies and tomato sauce wafted through the room, and my stomach clenched. I was very hungry. And optimistic.

"Mom should be back any minute now with our sodas," I said.

"Yeah, any minute," said Dad. "But we can go ahead and get started. Pizza's not good if it's cold."

We settled down and ate.

The minutes ticked by. Slowly. I didn't want to notice.

"Wonder where Mom is?" Rachel finally asked. "Do you think something happened?"

Mom had been gone almost an hour; it was unlike her to take so long.

"She might have met a friend and gotten into a long conversation," Dad said. He took a napkin from the coffee table and wiped his mouth.

"Why don't you call the store?" I asked. "They can tell you if she's still there."

"Good idea."

Dad went into the kitchen, where the phone was, and called. When he came back, his face was pale but his voice was calm. "They said she hasn't been there."

"Could she have gone to another convenience store?" I asked. There were several in our neighborhood.

Dad shook his head. "I don't know, Karena."

Rachel closed the pizza box. We had saved two pieces for Mom.

In the background, the movie continued with the character played by Tom Hanks asking the girl, played by Meg Ryan, if she wanted to meet at the top of the Empire State Building on Valentine's Day.

I had tears in my eyes from the movie. *If only life were like that,* I thought. *What a beautiful love story.*

Dad abruptly turned off the television. "I'm going to call your grandmother. Maybe she's heard from her."

Grammy also lived in Indianapolis, a few miles away. *Maybe she hitchhiked over there to get away from us for a while,* I thought. It sounded weird and illogical, but I was trying my best to come up with a reasonable explanation. Already, my stomach was twisting in knots.

When Dad came back from the kitchen, he shook his head. "Gram hasn't heard from her."

From that moment on, the night became one of numerous phone calls to the police and neighbors. To anyone who might have seen Mom.

Finally, after a couple of hours, Dad said, "Karena, you and Rachel go on up to bed. Mom will be back sometime tonight. And when you get up in the morning, she'll be at the breakfast table, explaining her adventure."

"Dad, do you think she left us?" Rachel asked. "You know . . . ran out on us?"

"She wouldn't leave us." I shook my head. "Momma wouldn't leave us."

"But you know how strange she's been lately." Rachel shot me a side glance. "And *mean.*"

"Girls, let's not get ahead of ourselves. I'm sure there's an explanation. I'm sure she's OK. She has to be. I'll deal with this. Best thing you can do is get some rest."

That's what adults always say when something is terribly wrong.

I looked at Dad, hoping I would be reassured by what I saw in his eyes.

But it wasn't good.

I knew things were not OK.

—

There was a constant rustling sound of the wind on the roof and in the trees. I crawled into bed and pulled up the old handmade patchwork quilt my babushka made for me when I was little. It provided some comfort and love. Something I'd been missing lately.

Twigs scratched noisily against the window, sounding like the claws of a monster who was trying to get inside. At twelve, I was still afraid to look outside at night. Too often, I'd seen red eyes staring back at me. Eyes from monsters. Vampires. Ghosts. I'd told Rachel over and over again that there were ghosts in the attic. I'd told her about the red eyes that stared at me from outside the window. But she told me I was just imagining things. Ever since Momma took us to see the movie *Poltergeist*, I'd been seeing the red eyes. And watching the tree limbs outside the window shake as if opening the portal to a supernatural world. I knew I was not imagining things, and I believed Rachel knew it too, because she was just as scared as I was. Neither one of us dared go into the attic. That door was inside our closet, and we both heard the ghosts all the time, skittering across the floor, bumping into things, knocking over things.

I had been having a recurring dream. It started with the headline of a movie, "Chapter One," popping up on the screen. Then a train traveled in a circle, and down below the railroad was a ditch, which was quite large. Below the ditch were caves and walkways and prisoners. In the train were vampires and ghosts. The train flew down the railroad tracks so fast, I had to hold on. I was barely hanging on to the outside of the train. I believed that if I jumped, I'd be safe, so I tried that, and occasionally I would land and be safe, but other times, I would get stuck inside the train and couldn't get out. Sometimes I would fall and die. Then I'd wake up.

I was not sure of it, but I believed this recurring dream was a reflection of my life. Like I was on a fast train and barely hanging on. I might survive. Or I might not.

In another dream, I was always at a movie theater. There was a closet at this theater, and I would go inside, and there were always vampires. Generally, I would fly out and escape the vampires, but sometimes I couldn't get out. I wondered if this was because Momma and I watched so many vampire movies like *The Lost Boys*. I enjoyed them a little bit, but when I went to bed, they haunted me.

I often thought that the red eyes I saw in my bedroom window were vampire eyes. As if they'd followed me out of my dream and into the real world. They scared me.

All of a sudden, the throbbing in my head was erratic and loud, and I was brought back to the situation at hand. Where was Momma?

Whispers flooded my ears, telling me that she was gone. But she couldn't be gone. She was just with us hours ago, telling us to order pizza and that she'd be back soon with sodas.

My stomach started to ache. Not from hunger but from the knowledge that things were not all right. My body was turning inside out, and I couldn't think straight.

Rachel and I shared a bedroom. We used to share a bed too, but not long before, Mom and Dad had let us choose separate beds. I chose a futon, and my sister chose a daybed. We split our room in half so we could feel like we had our own space. Above my dresser, I hung an oil painting I did of Momma in art class. She was a ghost, green like a zombie and wearing a white dress.

I couldn't go to sleep. My mind would not stop.

I had a musical pink teddy bear, and she was my favorite stuffed animal. I called her Bear. I got her when I was five, and she played "Somewhere Over the Rainbow" and "I'd Like to Teach the World to Sing (in Perfect Harmony)."

Rachel had a musical unicorn that she slept with that emitted a soft pale glow. I thought the unicorn protected her too.

I pulled back the covers, sat up in bed, and looked out the window, watching for Momma to come walking down the sidewalk. I didn't see red vampire eyes. I didn't see much of anything. More importantly, I didn't see Momma.

I felt an aloneness in my gut that I had never felt before. Our black cat, Keetska, which means "cat" in Ukrainian, scampered into my room. He was my only friend now and instinctively knew when I needed him. He jumped up on my bed, next to me and Bear, and started licking my face. I cuddled him close to me.

Moonlight pooled into the window from outside. I peered over at Rachel's side of the room, where lights and shadows splayed across the hardwood floor and up the wall.

"Sasha, are you asleep?" I still called her Sasha sometimes like I did when I was little at Babushka's, especially when I was afraid.

Rachel tossed and turned. "No."

"What do you think happened to Mom?"

"She probably met somebody at the store and went off with them."

"You mean like a boyfriend?" I was trying hard not to cry, but the tears rolled down my cheeks anyway, and I hugged my knees to my chest.

"Who knows? I don't care either way." Rachel's voice did not sound sad the way mine did.

"Don't say that, Rachel. She's our mom."

"She's been so mean to us lately, I don't care if she's gone. She doesn't give a shit about us, Karena."

"But she wouldn't leave us without saying goodbye, would she?" I was almost hysterical now. Frightened. I felt so alone. So small. So . . . abandoned.

"I don't know. Go to sleep, Karena. Close that curtain, will you? It's letting in too much light."

"I like watching for Mom."

"Look, Dad will find out what happened to her, and we'll know more tomorrow."

"OK. G'night, Sasha."

"G'night, Karena."

I turned from watching Rachel and looked out the bedroom window again. I saw a headlight approaching our house and held my breath. Did someone find Momma and bring her home to us?

When the car drove on by, I exhaled. I reached for the box of tissues on my nightstand and blew my nose. I could not stand the uncertainty. The not knowing.

A mourning dove began singing, "Whoooo-hoooo." Or was it an owl? Daddy said that everyone thought it was an owl, but really it was a mourning dove. The sweet song was so sad and sorrowful. As if the mourning dove already knew.

I couldn't sleep. I could not stop crying. Something in my life had changed. Something had shifted, and I was not sure what it was exactly. All I knew was that there was a deep aloneness, a void that could not be filled.

Things would never be the same again.

I knew this.

I thought back over the day's events. It had been a good day, right? I had been feeling a little bit hopeful, happy, and strong again. Mom hadn't talked about the devil at all in the past couple of days. Or about the fact that she thought Dad was the Antichrist.

How would we manage without her if she was really gone?

I was only twelve, certainly not old enough to look after Dad and Rachel or myself. And Rachel was only fourteen. She was not an adult yet either, even though she thought she was. How could she take care of us if Momma was gone? Daddy worked his day job as a therapist and had patients at the hospital at nighttime, and he played music with his band. And I didn't know what we were going to do.

Where was Mom?

Did she really meet someone at the store and run away? I had heard stories like that before. Maybe that's what happened.

Did she get kidnapped? Or was there something wrong inside Mom? That was it, I believed. I thought something terrible must be "inside" Mom. Some kind of poison that was destroying her. Some kind of demon. Some kind of evil, taking over.

Dear God, Mom wouldn't leave us, would she?

No, something really bad must have happened.

Mom must be dead.

"BEDROOM DYSMORPHIA"

Poem by Rachel Sahaidachny, 1993

Shadows creep through a placenta pink dream on
    air
as cold as ghosts' breath. Ice forms in twists on
    the windows.
Together, we whisper.
My sister tells me about red eyes in the window.
In the storm, the attic door tugs back and forth,
    shakes its frame.
We hug in our shared bed. The latch clicks,
the draft sucks the door in and out like a death
    rattle.
Our two sets of brown eyes stare at shadows on
    the wall.

The black pattern of tree limbs in dim light and
    folds in the curtains,
even the chest of drawers grows bigger, looks
    blacker,
a growing mass of blackness spreads to the bed.

We both know the portal to the other side.
Mother took us to see Poltergeist when I was five.
I recognize the cotton pink ectoplasm field
    asleep—pink foam
stuffed between old wooden boards,
pink as a ghost's womb.
In the furred layers of insulation
skeletons crack bones to discombobulate their
    joints.
Dolls trapped in bassinets become possessed,
their eyes glow fire, hair becomes static.
Old plush abandoned to collect dust comes to life,
    reaches out
from the black crack beneath the door.

CHAPTER TWELVE

When Love Goes Missing

Love . . . What is it, anyway?
Does it exist, or has it gone away?
Hate . . . It surrounds us everywhere.
It's something we must bear.
Life . . . What's the meaning of it?
There's no love in the world to count on . . .
Death . . . It strikes us in our mind
as something we must find . . .
But what we really need
is to find
love.

—Karena, age twelve

Vacant.

That's what her eyes looked like. *Vacant.* Deep blue that turned into an abyss of midnight, void of light. Void of identity, heart, warmth, love. That's what I saw in my recurring dreams about my mother. And that's what I saw when we found her.

The next morning, even before I opened my eyes, I knew something was wrong. *What was it? Oh, yes,* I remembered. Mom walked out of our house last night and didn't come back.

I rose up from my pillow, pushing Bear to the side, and looked out the window. It was a dark gray cloudy day. The kind of day that vampires would like. The wind blew through the tree branches, shaking the leaves until they fell to the ground in heaps of red and gold. I looked over to Rachel's side of the room and saw that she was already up, sheets and blankets left crumpled in a pile.

My heart leapt into my throat. *Did Mom come back last night?*

I jumped out of bed and ran downstairs in my pajamas. Eager. Hoping Mom would be sitting at the breakfast table, drinking a cup of coffee.

I bounded around the corner of the hallway and into the kitchen.

My heart stopped.

She was not there.

Rachel was in the kitchen, making toast. Dad sat there, drinking coffee, with a list of notes in front of him. Apparently, he had been writing down the places he had called.

"Dad, did you find Mom?"

He shook his head. "I drove around the neighborhood very early this morning and asked people if they had seen her . . . or anything suspicious. And some of the neighbors helped with the search too. No one saw anything, but they promised they would call if they heard any news."

"Did you talk to the police?" I asked, grabbing a mug and pouring myself a cup of coffee. Mom had told me I was too young to drink it, but from now on, I was going to drink coffee if I wanted to. Dad didn't seem to care one way or the other.

"I called them first thing this morning, and they don't know anything," Dad said.

"Want some toast?" Rachel mumbled. She had buttered several pieces, stacking them on a plate like pancakes. She seemed detached. I couldn't read her face and didn't know what she was thinking.

"Sure," I said. "Just one piece." Rachel handed me the plate piled with toast and put more bread into the toaster. As if she were an automated robot.

I was not so calm. My mind was racing. *Maybe someone kidnapped her, or worse. Maybe they killed her.* I didn't say this out loud, though. It sounded too surreal. Like something that happened to other people. Or on television shows. Not to people who lived in Indianapolis . . . or to my mother. Already, the very notion that Mom left us willingly was surreal enough.

"What about Grammy?" I asked, nibbling on a corner of the toast.

"I've been waiting to call her today," Dad said. "Hoping I'd have some good news for her. I scared her half to death last night."

"I don't think we'll find her," Rachel said. Her voice was full of gloom.

"Don't say that," I snapped. "There has to be a reasonable explanation."

The phone rang.

Dad jumped up and grabbed the receiver off the wall phone.

"Hello?" He held the phone out from his ear so Rachel and I could listen too.

"Nick, Linda is here with us," Grammy said.

"Oh, thank God," Dad said. "Rose, is she all right?" Rose was Grammy's name.

"Yes," Grammy said. "She's not hurt or anything. Seems to be fine. She walked most of the night, and when the cops picked her up, she told them to bring her here."

"Did she say why?"

"No, she didn't say much," Grammy said.

"OK, we're coming to get her right now," Dad said.

When Dad hung up, he looked at me and Rachel. "She walked all night long, and the police picked her up and took her to Grammy's."

"Why in the world would she do that?" Rachel asked.

"I don't know," Dad said. "C'mon, get your jackets. We'll go get her."

During the drive, we didn't talk much. We were all too numb.

When we arrived at Grammy's and she opened the front door, the combined scent of coffee and cinnamon greeted me. It was a familiar smell, one that I associated with Gram's home. One that I loved.

She hugged me and Rachel as we stood in the entryway. "She's in the kitchen."

"OK," Dad said.

"And Carol and Amanda are here too." Amanda was my cousin, Carol's daughter. "I called them last night and they drove up from Louisville. But, Nick, let's step into the living room first, before you go in there, and I'll brief you on what Linda told me about last night."

Dad swallowed hard. "Is . . . is she OK?"

Grammy nodded.

"Girls, why don't you all go on in and see your mother. I'll join you in a few minutes."

Rachel and I walked into the kitchen. We were nervous. Angry for what Mom had put us through last night but grateful she was OK. I just wanted her to come home with us and make everything all right in our house. *Normal.* I wanted *normal.*

Aunt Carol and Amanda stood at the stove, piling scrambled eggs and bacon on a platter. Hot cinnamon coffee cake sat on the counter. The smell was enticing and, for a moment, made me feel like all *was* normal.

At the kitchen table, there sat Mom, her hands around a cup of coffee. She looked strange. Different. Something was wrong with the way she looked at us. Something was wrong with her eyes. They seemed vacant. There was an emptiness, as if her soul had left. Or as if it had been hijacked by something evil.

Aunt Carol came over to me and Rachel and hugged us. "Oh, girls, so happy you're here."

"Hello, Rachel . . . Karena . . ." Mom's voice was detached, monotone. She acted as though everything was normal. But, of course, it wasn't.

Dad told me later what Grammy explained to him.

"Nick, I was going out of my mind when you told me Linda was missing last night." She folded and unfolded her hands, then wiped them on her apron. Her gray hair was frizzy and unkempt. *"I was frantic. And then when the cops called and told me they had found her wandering down the highway around two a.m., well, I was grateful she was alive. But I was furious that she had put us through hell, not knowing. And then when the cops dropped her off—Nick, she's been acting so strange. I was so worried, I called Carol, and she drove all the way from Louisville last night with Amanda to help us."*

"I'm just glad she had the police bring her here," Dad said. *"Honestly,*

she just told us she was going to the convenience store for some sodas. We had no idea anything was wrong."

Grammy nodded. "I know. I made breakfast for her—just some scrambled eggs and toast and some strawberries. But, Nick—she looked at it like it was poisoned. She barely took a bite. Afraid her own mother was trying to poison her. Can you imagine? I just don't know what to think."

"I know, Rose," he said. "She thinks everyone is out to get her right now. That we're all part of a satanic cult, part of the Antichrist movement or something."

Grammy looked at him with wide eyes. "Oh, Nick, you know about her father, right? He was a paranoid schizophrenic . . . and . . . and—"

"I know . . . I know."

"Evidently, Linda took out all her money from an ATM while she was walking and threw it in a ditch because she thought that the government put barcodes on the money and could track her electronically. She said something about learning this through her studies on the New World Order. Then she tossed her driver's license into the ditch so nobody could identify her."

"Her paranoia has been building," Dad said. "Was she at all coherent when the police dropped her off?"

"Yes, oddly so," said Gram. "She mentioned that a man stopped his car and walked toward her once, and she just started yelling at him to go away. Then she laughed and said that he probably thought she was crazy."

"Did she say anything about God or the devil telling her to do that last night?" Dad asked.

"She mumbled something about being so full of sin that she was turning very dark. She said she had a Bible with her and got tired and stopped at a church—St. John's, I think—and rested awhile. She was far past the county line at this point."

"She probably thought a saint would come and rescue her if she was sitting in a church," Dad said. "Good God."

"When the police dropped her off, she was limping and her shin was swollen. I don't know if she fell or what, but her clothes were soiled and she had dirt on her face."

Dad's voice got quiet. "Rose, I don't know what to do."

"She needs help, Nick," Gram said. "I wish I had gotten help when I learned how sick her father was, but those were different times. I thought I had to be a good wife and accept what God had given me."

"We all do the best we can," Dad said sympathetically.

"When the police found her, she told them that the demons were coming for her, but she was hoping the Lord showed up first. They brought her some hot chocolate, but she was afraid to drink it, afraid they had drugged it. After they coaxed her for a while, she told them to bring her here, thank heavens. We cleaned her up a little, and she slept for a while on the couch. She told us not to call you until today. I called as soon as I could."

Dad just shook his head.

"Nick, she is broken. Whatever is wrong with her, she is broken. Like pieces of glass. And she is very mad at you, you know."

"I know," Dad said. "She doesn't trust me because she believes I'm part of the Antichrist. It's bad, Rose, really bad. I need to see her."

"Go on in there . . . She's in the kitchen."

When Dad walked into the kitchen, Mom looked up nonchalantly, as if it were just another morning. "Hi, Nick."

"Hello, Linda. You had us scared half to death. The girls were worried out of their minds."

His jaw was clenched, which meant he was furious as hell.

Mom shrugged. *Didn't she care that we had been worried?* She wore a baggy sweater that Gram had given her. She had on the same jeans that she was wearing when she left the house, but they were stained and torn, as if she had rolled down a hill. Her shoulder-length brown hair hung in tangles. She looked as though she had aged ten years since she'd left our house. And she acted like we were strangers.

This mother was not the mother that Rachel and I had known all our lives. And even though we had witnessed some strange behavior from Mom lately, the person in front of us seemed like someone else.

Rachel and I stood by, just staring, not knowing what to say to her.

"C'mon, get your things. We're going home." Dad's voice was stern. Firm.

Mom nodded and got up from the table.

"Nick, why don't you and the girls stay and have some breakfast?" Gram said. "You don't have to hurry home."

"I think we should go."

Aunt Carol and Amanda hovered nearby but said nothing.

Gram walked over to Mom. "Linda, are you going to be all right?"

"Sure. I'm fine."

"Where are the rest of your clothes? Your purse?" Dad ran his fingers through his hair.

"I'll show you," Mom said. "They're in an area by a river I passed where I threw out my personal things."

Dad looked at the floor, and for a moment, he seemed speechless. Then he turned to Gram. "Thanks, Rose, for everything."

Gram hugged all of us. Aunt Carol and Amanda hugged us too. We all had tears in our eyes. None of us knew exactly what we were dealing with. But we all knew something momentous had just happened.

I felt a gnawing in my stomach. A craving or hunger that would not be satiated for a long, long time.

This was the first time Mom disappeared from our home. It was the first time she ran away from us, but it wouldn't be the last.

PART THREE

Sinner

CHAPTER THIRTEEN

Do the Birds Still Sing in Hell?

Bring me freedom, send me death,
suck away my forsaken breath.
This love cuts deep
(into my veins).
You made me lie.
(A sinner, am I?)

—Karena, age twelve

Drama.

It felt as though this was what it was all about. Mom's love for drama. Her way to get attention from Dad. What else could it be? Mom was always screaming to me and Rachel about Dad and all his faults. She was paranoid and jealous, convinced Dad was having an affair. She was mistrusting and delusional and declared that a satanic group was monitoring us through the television set. And she was convinced that people whom Dad worked with were all in on the satanic conspiracy.

For me, it was all hell.

For a while, I tried to think the best, even though I felt scared and abandoned. But when she left us, it shook me. Why had she taken off and gone to Gram's without letting us know where she was going? *Who does that?* Momma surely wouldn't disappear from our home and stay out the entire night if she loved us, would she? Didn't she know how worried we would all be? How scared Rachel and I would be?

But there were times Momma could act normal, like a regular mom. And those were the times that pulled me in. Rachel, on the other hand, didn't believe that everything was going to be all right.

—

On the way from Grammy's, Mom directed Dad to a riverbank where she said she had thrown away her purse, her driver's license, and her wedding ring. We all got out of the car and scoured the area but couldn't find anything.

"It probably washed away in the river," Dad said.

"I'm sure this is where I threw out my things," she said.

I didn't know whether to believe her.

The rest of the drive home felt like it was taking us to the other side of the earth. None of us knew what we were driving back to. Would Mom return to the person she had been? One who could be creative and sweet? Or would she remain distant, detached, and cold?

Rachel and I rode in the back seat and Mom up front with Dad. We were quiet. We didn't know what to say. I just wanted to feel my mother's arms embracing me. The thought brought tears to my eyes. I tried to push the feeling of needing her far out of my mind.

Who was this strange woman coming home with us? What had happened to her?

There was nothing lonelier than what I felt on that warm fall day, riding in a car with a family that seemed cut off from the world. Everything felt dull. Now and then, a blast of color from the autumn foliage would pierce the scene, and the sunlight was so crystal and brilliant, it made me ache. For beauty. For normalcy. For regular parents.

I kept trying to resist the thought, but on some level, I knew that life would never be the same. Not for me, Rachel, Dad, or Mom. Not for Grammy or Aunt Carol. Not for any of us.

Something had broken in our family, and each one of us was forever scarred and changed. Our lives had been shattered into a million pieces of jagged glass. I knew that no matter how hard any of us tried, we'd never be able to glue the pieces back together again.

When we got home, Mom said she needed rest and flew up the stairs as light streamed through the stained glass window on the landing.

Dad told us not to worry. "Just give her some time. She'll be fine, I hope."

"But, Dad, what happened?" I finally spoke up after Mom was upstairs. "Did Gram tell you? Did Rachel and I do something wrong?"

"She just needed some time to herself," Dad said. "It's not your fault, Karena. It's not Rachel's fault, or my fault. She just felt the need to get away for a while."

"I don't trust her," Rachel said.

"She'll be all right now," I said, trying to reassure Rachel . . . and myself. "Maybe Dad's right. Maybe she just needed some time alone."

"I don't believe that for one second. And neither should you!" Rachel shook her head and stomped upstairs.

"I'm going into the office for a bit," Dad said. "I'll stop and get some food for us when I come back. I won't be gone long."

"OK," I said.

With Dad gone and Mom and Rachel in their bedrooms, I was alone. But I didn't know how to handle the feelings I was experiencing. Mom had rejected us the night before. She had just walked out. *Normal people didn't do that, did they?* She couldn't love us, or she wouldn't have left us. I couldn't trust her anymore, and I hated everything about my life at that moment.

Sitting in the living room alone, all I could think about was escaping this world. Nothing seemed right or normal. And I didn't feel loved or wanted. I felt like I had no purpose. I couldn't bear the thought of another day. My life was hell, and I was only twelve years old. I simply didn't want to live anymore.

I believed that suicide was a sin. That's what they'd taught us at church. That you would go to hell if you killed yourself. But I didn't care. I was a sinner, anyway, and it didn't matter anymore. I wasn't sure what hell would be like, if there were animals there or other people, if there were hummingbirds or mockingbirds that sang, but it had to be better than where I was on earth. On earth, I was already in hell.

Feeling nothing at all would be better than this pain that was quickly consuming me.

CHAPTER FOURTEEN

Dripping Blood

If I could just find some slivers of hope,
I believe I could live with this pain.
I believe I could forget that I want to die.
I believe I could forget how good it feels to cut
and see the red bubbles in my bath.
But I need those slivers of hope
and I cannot find them.

—Karena, age twelve

Crimson bubbles.

It had been a week since Mom disappeared from our home.

I turned on the faucet and began to fill the bathtub with water. I wanted it to be hot. So hot that it would almost burn me so I would become numb and wouldn't feel the pain. Next, I poured in some lavender bubble bath. Bubbles would be good. Dad had bought those for me and Rachel, thinking that we would enjoy bubble baths. Thinking that, perhaps, Mom would enjoy a bubble bath every now and then too.

Barefoot, I walked over the cold tiled floor to the bathroom sink and picked up Dad's razor from the glass container beside his bottle of shaving cream. It was not a disposable razor but one of those old-fashioned ones. I opened the razor and carefully took out the blade, shiny and new. *Good.* That meant it was sharp. Really sharp. He had probably just put it in that morning. He didn't like it if us girls used his razor to shave our legs. He said it made the blade dull. But he wouldn't think about that afterward . . . *if I went through with it.* I placed the razor on the bathtub's edge, then ran my fingers through the water. Hot and steamy and bubbly. *Good.* I took off my clothes, piled them in a heap on the floor, and slid into the bathwater. It smelled heavenly . . . just like lavender flowers, and the heat stung my skin.

The bubbles rose and covered my waist and then my chest, and I slipped down further, my long hair floating like weeds. I let all the pain escape to the surface. The water was so soothing. Even exhilarating.

I'll just do it a little, I told myself. *Just enough to see what it feels like. Just enough to see if it changes the pain.*

I took the razor blade and touched it to the skin on my palm. And then I dragged it across my palm, slicing it. *Just a little.* A tingle arced across my scalp. And I felt happy.

Then another little cut . . . *just a little* . . . and a perfect straight line of blood bloomed from under the edge of the blade. I watched, mesmerized, as the line grew into a long, round bubble. A lush crimson bubble that got bigger and bigger. *Crimson bubbles.* Shiny. Sparkly. Beautiful. Could be a title someone might use for a song.

I closed my eyes. It didn't hurt. Not really.

That's when I knew it would be so easy. So easy to cut another line . . . and another . . . until I just drifted down into the water and away from this world. No more pain. No more disappointments. No more heartache.

I held my hand up and dripped blood into the bathwater. More crimson bubbles clustered together.

Somewhere outside, a dog barked, and I heard a horn honk as a car drove by. Probably warning the dog to get out of the street.

I sank further into the water and closed my eyes. My mind drifted to when I first woke up that morning. Rachel was still in bed. She usually slept in way past me. It was mainly because she hid in the closet reading most of the day and into the night and was tired in the mornings.

I was born at the break of dawn. I was often the first one up, and

I'm like that to this day. My middle name is Dawn, and perhaps my parents named me that because, intuitively, they knew I would be a morning person.

Since it was Sunday, the day stretched out long and lonesome before me. I looked out the window above my bed. It was a cloudy, drizzly morning. I noticed that all the blinds were pulled down on the neighbors' houses. It felt like they were keeping themselves shielded from our house. From our secrets. Our pain. Our worries. Our neighbors knew that something was not right on our street. They had tried to help us find Mom. They had witnessed the fear in our eyes. I thought they knew there were monsters lurking in our home. Even though we'd hidden it well for a long time, the truth was now out.

Mom had been home for over a week after disappearing that night, but she didn't seem to be getting any better. She stayed in her room most of the time, and Dad was often out. That left me and Rachel alone for the most part, to tend to ourselves. And since Rachel either kept to herself most of the time or hung out with her friends, it meant that I was mostly by myself.

My soul had been dying just a little bit more every day. When I was at school, I wandered aimlessly through the crowded hallways to my locker. I wanted to hide in there. I couldn't talk to anyone about what was happening at home. I had tried to talk to my girlfriends, Emma and Megan, about my mom's problems, but they looked at me like I was weird or crazy. My girlfriends didn't understand. So I pretended everything was OK so my friends would think I was happy and normal.

Ironically, while my mom became a religious fanatic, I was starting to doubt that there was a God. I used to believe in God. I even gave sermons to our family in the living room on Sundays, whether we attended church services or not. Dad bought a Casio keyboard for me, and I would play it and act like I was performing in church. But as Mom started abandoning us, it felt like God was leaving my side too.

So I was on my own. Just me and my journal.

—

One thing that particularly bothered me was that Mom was destroying her beautiful artwork in the house and in the art room in the basement even more frequently. She had painted a gorgeous large oil painting of a dahlia flower that hung at the entry of the house. I came home from school one day and saw that she had ripped it into pieces and burned it in the fireplace.

"Momma," I cried, "why did you burn your beautiful painting?"

"Oh, Karena," she said. "Don't you know? If you own or wear a *graven image*, that means you are against God since you're worshipping an image."

I did not understand. The words sounded foreign.

And though I didn't think things could get any worse, they did. Rachel and I were no longer allowed to wear any clothes with images. And we couldn't watch television or listen to music. It was a form of demonic temptation, Mom told us. We couldn't even use cash anymore because of the images of the presidents on the bills. When we needed to use cash, she would scratch out the presidents' faces.

Our home became increasingly strange. Stale. Empty. Void of life or warmth. Void of love. It was during the week after her disappearance that I first began to think about suicide.

My agitation increased with Mom's agitation, which increased Dad's agitation. He tried to get Mom to seek medical help, but she refused.

"Your father is in a satanic cult, Karena," Mom spat at me one night while Dad was off playing music again. "He's a cheat, a liar, and a satanist. You can't believe anything he tells you, and you cannot trust him."

The truth was, I didn't know what or whom to believe. Mom was very good at persuading me at times that Dad was the enemy. For a while, I hated Dad, thinking that maybe it was his fault that Mom had changed so dramatically.

Later—much later—Dad explained that schizophrenia can take off into religiosity, but it's a simulated delusional system.

When she started changing, I didn't know the medical terms for Mom's mental problems. All I knew was that she was broken, Dad was broken, and our entire family was broken.

I was extremely unhappy and torn between my mother and father. I wanted to trust and love both of them. I wanted both of them to trust and love me, but most of the time, I felt alone and unloved.

—

"I can't stay here anymore," Mom said one night a year or two after she'd first disappeared. She and Dad had been screaming at each other for more than an hour.

"Fine!" Dad yelled. "Why don't you go to your mother's house for a few days? Would do you some good."

"No." There was ice in her voice. "You're not hearing what I'm saying. I need to *leave*. Move out."

For a moment, Dad just stood there with his mouth open. I was sitting on the top landing of the stairs, my stomach knotted up again, listening to their fight and hoping that they would make up. But I knew they wouldn't.

"Where will you go?" Dad asked.

"I need to be on my own awhile. I already got an apartment, and I have a new job I'm starting next week with a maid service. It's a reputable company."

Dad looked shocked again. Mom was a trained social worker and had always done well at her places of employment. She was exceptionally good at pretending that she was normal.

Why in the world would she want to work as a maid when she had a career as a social worker?

"What about the girls?" he asked.

"They can come and visit me in my apartment, or I can stop by here and visit them. I have my car. I just need to be on my own for a while."

"OK, Linda," Dad said after a moment of silence. "If this is what you need."

I was quiet. Even though I wanted to scream, *Mom, please don't leave us!* I didn't. I knew it wouldn't do any good.

So Mom packed a few things and left that evening.

"Mom is gone," I said out loud when Rachel and I went to bed later that night. "I can't believe it. She is officially gone."

I hugged my stuffed animal, Bear, and my cat, Keetska, and started crying.

"Why are you crying?" Rachel asked. "She said we could visit her on weekends, and she'd come and see us. To tell you the truth, I'm happy about it. I don't really want to see her. She has always been worse to me than she has to you. In fact, she's been outright brutal toward me. I can never do anything right. I'm not even allowed to have friends. And you know that's true, Karena. She puts me down every time she can. Even when I won awards for the short stories that I wrote, Mom criticized me and said they weren't very good. I can never, ever do anything to satisfy her."

"But, Rachel, she's gone . . . really *gone!*" I grabbed a Kleenex from the box by my bed and blew my nose.

"And don't forget how she accused both of us of stealing her ideas when we paint. Instead of telling us how beautiful our artwork was, she screamed at us that we're thieves. Also, I have no privacy. She even went through my dresser drawers to find my notes and journals to use things I wrote in them against me. She said I was evil. So, no, I'm not unhappy that she's gone."

"She said all of us were evil," I said. "Not just you."

"Don't you remember that I had to throw my journals out finally because I was afraid that she would read them? I don't know what she thought she was going to find. She was determined to prove that I was a witch or evil in some way. And when she realized she couldn't control me any longer, she became even more abusive."

"But, Rachel, she's our mother!" I hugged Bear tighter.

Couldn't Rachel understand what was happening? We were still kids. We did not know how to live in a household or go about our days without our mom. Especially with Dad gone so often.

"You'd better be careful, Karena," Rachel warned. "She's abusive to you all the time too, and you don't even realize what's happening because you're still too young and you believe that everything is going to be all right. So just be careful."

Rachel turned the light out beside her bed. "G'night, Karena. Trust me, this is best for all of us."

"Night, Sasha," I said.

I curled up in a fetal position with Bear and continued to cry. It was actually more than crying. It was the kind of desolate sobbing that comes from a person drained of all hope. My breathing was ragged, gasping.

I cried until no more tears came, but the emptiness and sorrow remained.

After my mom moved out, I took more hot bubble baths and continued to experiment with cutting myself *just a little*. When I went to school, I wore long sleeves so no one could see the cuts on my arms. It empowered me, made me feel like I was in control of *something, anything*, when everything else was chaos. When I cut myself, the sharpness of the blade distracted me from the sharp pain in my heart.

The dripping blood—the *crimson bubbles*—became more and more irresistible.

CHAPTER FIFTEEN

Darkness and Friends

Why must the world be so sad?
Why can't we forgive each other?
Why can't we all love each other?
Why are you lying to me?
Why are you crying so painfully in my ear?
Why should I care?

—Karena, age thirteen

Old friend.

I've known darkness for a long time. Darkness felt like a friend.

At nighttime, darkness can make the streets look like an old-fashioned photograph . . . everything a shade of light and gray. But inside a person's soul, darkness becomes something else. It can rob you of your best self and replace it with fear. Or surrender. Or rebellion. In this type of darkness, I have lingered often, muscles cramped and unable to move. In my life, there have been many sides of darkness . . . many shades of light and gray.

When something is with you long enough, though, it can become your friend while also being your enemy. In this way, darkness became a friend. And when I was a child, even when the night sky bore no stars, or the moon didn't shine, darkness was there for me.

—

The paralyzing pain crept through my body. I tried to ignore it. Once I slipped into the crimson bubbles, the hurt would ooze into the water along with the blood.

I had to face the truth. The reality that Mom had officially left us. Dad tried to soften the blow by telling me and Rachel that Mom was trying to work through some stuff. She would be back when she was ready. But aside from occasional visits, she stayed away through my preteen and teenage years. Dad tried hard to maintain a sense of normalcy in our home, but it didn't feel normal at all to me.

At fourteen, I poured my feelings into my journal, writing entries like this:

> *I am so sad! It is January and it is snowing. The air is delicate and cold. It dances on my skin like icy waves on a winter's beach. Everything is washed in hues of gray, and a murky light settles on the trees and houses all around me. As I walk home from school, I look down and watch my boots moving over the frozen sidewalk, perfect concrete slabs, flat and square, and in other moments, my eyes are transfixed to the interplay of cloud and sun above.*
>
> *I am in high school and should be enjoying this time, but I am too unhappy. My world is too dark. Mom has been gone for months now. Rachel and I have been to visit her apartment on weekends, and it's a hollow place. There is no furniture. She sleeps on a blanket on the hard wooden floor and calls it her home. There is little heat on these cold, cold nights. There are no lamps. She only has candles for light. She says that she likes to eat by candlelight. Rachel and I do not know what she's eating. There are empty cans of tuna fish.*

Empty boxes of crackers. Mom does come over to our
house to visit and stay with us sometimes. But her love
for us is not real.
    I am so sad.

—

To cope, along with the cutting in the bathtub, which started when I was twelve, I became obsessed with getting high on pot and on Ecstasy, or E, as everyone at school called it. Dad didn't have a clue. But I loved both of these drugs. E was an especially wild, wonderful escape!

I also skipped school all the time to meet friends behind old buildings downtown and get high. My drug use continued through high school. By the age of fifteen, I was doing every street drug I could get my hands on—marijuana, crack, cocaine, quaaludes, meth, and every hallucinogen in between. I couldn't think about anything else. I'd go home for dinner and be sitting there at the kitchen table, flying high. Nobody knew the extent of what I was doing except for Rachel. Sometimes I'd laugh and tell her, "I'm high, but don't tell anyone."

For all I knew, Rachel was high too. Neither one of us could deal with what was happening in our family. My attitude sucked. I became reckless and didn't care about anyone or anything. I simply wanted to party and get high.

Tattoos were another way I coped. At sixteen, I got my first tattoo on my lower back; it stands for "eternity—eternal life." Later, at eighteen, when I was living in LA, I got a tattoo of the Japanese symbol for strength and power. It still comforts and empowers me to this day whenever I look at it. It has become my daily reminder that I can be strong and survive anything. That I have the power inside me to overcome.

Japanese symbol for strength and power

But when I was still in high school, after the first tattoo, I got pierc-
ings on my tongue and belly button. I hid these from my parents and
relished in the secrecy of it.

—

In high school, all I wanted to do was hide the pain inside me and
rebel. Do drugs. Eventually, have sex.

Dad urged me to talk to a counselor at school, so I went to see the
only one we had, Mr. James. A dull, uninspiring man who wore wire-
rimmed glasses and had a bushy black mustache that overwhelmed his
small, angular face. He was clueless.

I sat across the desk from him, my body slumped in the chair and
my legs sprawled in front of me. Very tomboyish. *I don't have time for
this,* I told myself.

"What's going on with you, Karena?" he asked.

"I don't know what you're talking about," I said, sniffing.

Mr. James stared at me as if I were a hopeless delinquent. *Don't you
know the hell I'm going through at home?* I wanted to scream at him.
*Don't you know my mom hates me? And Dad is about as clueless as
they come? Don't you know anything, Mr. James?*

But I didn't. I just grinned and jutted out my chin like a haughty
Miss Know-It-All.

"Karena, are you doing drugs?" Mr. James was direct. "Is that why
you're skipping school so much? Are you on drugs right now?"

I stared out the window, squinting my eyes at the sunlight streaming through, and ignored him.

"Look, I know you're going through a rough time," he said. His
voice was soft and soothing, but there was no way I was going to open
up to this pseudo-therapist about anything. "I know this can't be easy,"
he continued. "Your mom and all. Well, I understand."

You don't know anything! You can't possibly understand, I screamed
inwardly. I wanted to show him the scars on my arms from my cutting
and shout at him, *Look at this! Do you know what this feels like?*

"Look, I have to get to my next class." I was done. I refused to tell
him anything.

"Come back anytime if you want to talk," Mr. James said.

It was a dull visit.

Afterward, Mr. James called Dad and told him that he should take me to a real therapist. I needed lots of help.

Dad called Mom and told her what Mr. James said. Surprisingly, after she heard this, she came over to the house one night. At first, Dad downplayed the whole therapist idea, though. "After all, I'm a therapist myself," he said, "and I think Karena will be OK."

I thought Mom would be sympathetic, but she made it about her.

"She's wild, Nick. She needs some discipline."

She turned to me next. "Karena, you're always getting into trouble, and you're turning into a real delinquent. You're embarrassing me."

What? I'm *embarrassing* her?

I just stared at her.

This wasn't the first time she turned things on me. For a while, whenever Mom dropped by our home, she would yell at me for what seemed like hours.

"How could you do this to me, Karena? You're making me look like a fool with skipping school and doing God knows what!"

"Linda, that's enough," Dad chimed in.

"I . . . I . . . I didn't do anything to you, Mom," I said. Even though I tried my best to not cry, tears were spilling onto my cheeks.

"You're only doing this for attention, Karena. You're embarrassing me and your father in front of all the teachers and students, and our neighbors, and you should be ashamed of yourself."

Mom's hair was tied back from her face, and she was still wearing her house-cleaning uniform. I noticed that her fingernails were ragged, her hands wrinkled from cleaning with bleach all day. She almost seemed like her normal self, except that other "normal" Mom would have never let her fingernails look ragged. She used to be so concerned with her looks. And the "other" Mom would have been kinder to me.

I shrugged. "I'm all right. I feel fine. I do not need to see a therapist."

At that point, I got up from the kitchen table and ran out of the house to find my friends so I could get high. I could not bear to be in that house any longer with my mentally ill mother accusing me of embarrassing *her.*

I learned how to keep quiet about my issues. I learned how to not cry. I knew Mom was mentally off-balance, but she often made me feel like a mentally ill person myself. So I learned to keep it all inside. *Do not let anyone see the pain.*

But I was overwhelmed by sadness. The veil of darkness was thick, heavy, and smothering.

—

During high school, I frequently stayed over at the homes of my girl-friends Megan and Emma. I often didn't bother to come home for dinner after school, and I wouldn't call Dad to let him know where I was. I just couldn't bear the thought of going home. I knew that Dad would drive around the streets at night, looking for me. I simply didn't care. Sometimes he'd pass me smoking pot on a street corner with my friends. But whenever I saw his car, I'd run and hide. I didn't want to go home.

Megan and Emma helped me through this dark, sad time. We'd go to the White River, nestled in a wooded area about a mile from my house, and sit on the beach in front of a big oak tree. We painted the trees around this area to give it a more colorful look, and wrote down thoughts, dreams, and notes on pieces of paper, which we then buried in the dirt beneath the trees. We called the place at the river the Painted Memories Beach, or PMB, for short. We even dug for treasure, thinking that someone might have hidden gold or maps there. We'd wade along the edge of the river, getting covered in mud and decaying leaves. It didn't matter to us that the river could be dangerous or that there was broken glass and all kinds of debris in the water. It was the place that held our secrets and our dreams. It was the place that witnessed our fears and pain. It was our sanctuary away from hard reality. Even though Megan and Emma weren't experiencing the same kind of pain I was, they liked to escape their everyday worlds too.

It was also the place where I immersed myself in some of my darkest thoughts. I would sit on the riverbank by myself and stare into the water. I was lonely and starved for warmth. For love, really. The sounds of nature kept me company when no one was around; this was where I first found comfort in nature. Sometimes my breathing would become erratic, deep or shallow. Fear sat quietly within me. I fought it.

I would sit alone on the damp ground, feeling the frigid water from the river's edge seep into my jeans. With my hands resting on the soil and my back to the oak tree, I remained, waiting, breathing . . . wondering how I could make it through another day. I noticed that if you followed the water as it meandered through dark, spiderwebbed culverts, you'd find gnarled, lightning-blasted cedars and thick pines. A place where memories could hide and secrets could be buried.

At Painted Memories Beach, I found some semblance of peace. Sitting on the riverbank, listening to the chirping of crickets and songbirds, the bad memories could disappear downstream, washed away over the rocks by thoughts of happier times. Sometimes, when I was wading through my memories, I found the jagged pieces of myself had been broken and strewn haphazardly everywhere, tossed casually inside that deep, dark forest.

Later in life, I realized that when I went to PMB, I was subconsciously excavating the pieces and trying to put myself back together again. The excavating, the careful and most assuredly painful retrieval and polishing of the tiny pieces, could help make me whole again. *Almost.*

Looking back, I wonder if any of us who have been abandoned by a parent or lost a loved one due to mental illness, or experienced something similarly devastating, can ever really be whole again. The best we can do is trudge onward like little soldiers, hoping that tomorrow will be a better day. That tomorrow there will be rays of sunshine we can revel in, that tomorrow there will be a little bit of happiness in our mostly gray world. Sometimes the sunshine is there. And sometimes it is not.

Even at the young age of fourteen, I grappled with this—the reality of trudging onward, the search for hope, and what to do when you can't find it. Again, I turned to my journal.

> *I cannot stand this! I need a gun to make everything better. I just keep telling myself to hold on . . . just hold on . . . and things will get better. I try to appear calm, but inside I am screaming. I need to escape from here. It's impossible to sleep at home. The red vampire eyes in my bedroom window . . . the ghosts in my attic . . .*

the anger and hate that spreads out and climbs up the walls.

Tears trickle down my face. I am so sick of crying. The tears drip in my mouth and I taste the saltiness. I wish I had a normal life. A normal mother and father who loved each other and who loved me and Rachel. But the world is so twisted. It's insane, just like everyone in it.

Every time Mom gets me in a room alone, she tells me that Dad is in a cult, and that this cult is going to take her away. And the cult will come after me when I grow up. I am suspicious of everyone and have no one I can trust. Mom says the people in these cults are wonderful liars. And these liars are everywhere. At church. At school. Where Dad works. They're part of the Antichrist, she says. They act like Christians, but they're twisting things around, tricking you into believing their own warped notions. Mom says that I am the only person she can trust. But who can I trust?

I have been painting, and that, along with the cutting, the E, and everything else, is the only way I can cope. Most of the time. But I am so tired of this. I am in so much pain.

That's it. I will just have to leave soon. I hope . . . well, I will try to think happy thoughts until then. I will try to lock away the pain and smile and act like everything is OK.

I know it is not.

CHAPTER SIXTEEN

When the Vampires Sank Their Fangs into My Soul

Look out the window
See the sun shining
Why can't it shine on me?
Really not needed . . . So why am I here?
A figure in the background
that no one sees.
Isolate myself . . . curl up and die.
Should anyone care?
Don't worry.
No use in trying to be happy.
No use in hiding my feelings.
If I slip out till no existence,
and cry in a dark room . . .
Would anyone realize? Would anyone care?
Father can't love me; he's just a liar . . .
Mother can't love me; I don't believe in her "God."
Sister just hates me, and everyone else . . .
Friends can't guess who's the best.
Believe in myself, it's all I can do.
Love who I must love . . . oh, very few.
Take a drug to calm me down.

For now, can't wait until I die.
Erase my fears . . . How can I? Impossible.
Cry no more tears . . . How can I? Impossible.
But I can try, yes, I'll try . . . Until the time when I
     can die.

—Karena, age thirteen

Am I dead?
Is this what death feels like?
Did the vampires finally sink their fangs into my soul?
And rip out my heart?
What is going on?
Everything feels so strange.
For a moment, I didn't feel a thing. I was just floating. And it was kind of blissful. I lingered in between sleep and consciousness. A twilight world. I did not see any vampires, so I must have escaped them.

Then I heard a beeping sound like one of those monitors in a hospital. I started to zone out again. If I was not dead, then what happened?

I felt someone's fingers pick up my wrist. It must be a nurse? I believed she was checking my pulse, and I heard her say, "She should wake up soon."

Everything was fuzzy. This must be a hospital, but I didn't know exactly where I was. I was confused. A tiny bit of fear tortured my guts, churning my stomach in tense cramps. This fear engulfed my consciousness, knocking all other thoughts aside.

I heard my parents crying over my bed. *Good God, I believe Mom is praying to Jesus.*

Before I opened my eyes, I knew there were bright lights in the room because I could feel them on my eyelids.

My memory scrolled through the data in my brain. What happened?

Oh yeah, Megan and I were at Emma's house. Her parents were out having dinner, and it was just us three girls there. It was a Saturday night, and we were in the basement, listening to CDs, talking about boys, and drinking Captain Morgan's rum. At first, we mixed it with soda, but eventually I started drinking it straight from the bottle. We just wanted to get drunk and smoke cigarettes.

One cool thing about being at Emma's was her mother's medicine cabinet. She was a nurse and always had bottles and bottles of pills. Uppers and downers. Painkillers. Anything, really, that anyone could want.

That night, I was depressed and tired from all the chaos in my life. I teetered between wanting to numb the pain and wanting to make sure I would never feel it again.

At one point, I took the bottle of Captain Morgan's and went upstairs into Emma's mom's bedroom. I opened the medicine cabinet and took out several bottles of pills. I thought these pills were magical and would be a great way to get rid of the pain inside. I had made up my mind: I wanted to die.

"Karena! Karena! Can you hear me?" I later recalled Emma screaming at me, then shouting at Megan to help her get me up off the ground. I also remembered lying curled up on the floor and throwing up all over everything.

Then, Emma and Megan were pulling my arms and dragging me into the shower, clothes and all. Cold water splashing on me; mascara running down my cheeks, burning my eyes; Emma crying. The awful bile in my throat, the churning of my stomach, and the shower soaking me to the bone.

And then, after I was thoroughly drenched, they dragged me out. Somebody took off my wet clothes and dressed me in Emma's sweatpants and sweatshirt. I curled up into a ball, and next thing I knew, Mom was holding me like she did when I was a baby.

Evidently, someone had called my parents. I remembered Mom crying. I told her, "I'm going to heaven to be with Jesus."

—

I had taken a handful of pills because I wanted to kill myself. One of my friends called 911 and then called my parents. I learned the medics had pumped my stomach as I lay on the floor at my friend's house. Later, the doctors said I had lost my pulse for a moment.

We all wish life were a dream—the dreams where the sky is blue, flowers are blooming, the sun is shining, and the happy people are smiling. But then, you wake up from "the Land of Perfect Happiness," and you begin to cry. But why? Then you realize you're not alone. Everyone is sad. Hidden behind their smiles, there's hatred. No one lives a perfect life. We all think once or twice about ending it. We all think about holding the pill and tipping the glass. And fading into a perfect sleep . . . forever. Some of us go through with it. Some of us don't because we know there's something in life that we are waiting for . . . or maybe there's a light somewhere that gives us hope. Some of us are too scared, some try to run away from their pain, but there's no use . . . 'cause your problems are there, always . . . waiting.

—

The heart monitor beeped loudly.

My eyelids fluttered open.

Mom and Dad were both crying over my bed.

"Look! She's awake," Dad said. "Karena, can you hear me?"

My mouth felt like there was a wad of cotton in it. There was some kind of tube down my throat, which was uncomfortable.

"I need some water," I said out of the side of my mouth. My voice sounded hoarse. Dry. Raw. I was so thirsty.

"Oh, Karena, you're awake!" Mom cried.

"I don't know if I can give you water," Dad said. "You have a tube down your throat."

A doctor came into my room. "Oh, good, she's awake." He looked at me. "Karena, do you remember who the president is?"

"Ronald Reagan." I didn't know why I said that, because I knew exactly who the president was and it certainly was *not* Ronald Reagan. Not sure if I was trying to be funny or what.

They all chuckled. That relieved me. I didn't want to see them worrying or in pain.

"She's thirsty," Dad said.

"Let's give her some orange juice," the doctor said. "I'll take out the tube."

It hurt when he pulled out the tube, and I gagged. Then the doctor poured some orange juice from a pitcher into a plastic cup, put a bendy straw in it, and let me take a sip. "Go slow," the doctor said. "Just a little."

I wanted to guzzle the entire cup of juice, but my throat was so raw, I could only manage a few sips of it.

"How are you feeling?" the doctor asked.

"I'm OK." I struggled to sit up.

"Do you know what happened?" He held my chart in his hands, reviewing my vitals.

"I . . . I . . . My friends and I got drunk, and . . . I took some pills." I shot a look at Mom and Dad, knowing they would disapprove. I wasn't sure whether they knew I had been trying to kill myself.

The doctor nodded and adjusted his eyeglasses. "Well, you were lucky, young lady. You vomited most of the pills before you passed out, which probably saved your life."

I just stared at him. *What did he want me to say?*

I had a catheter in that was beginning to feel extremely uncomfortable. I squirmed a bit in bed.

"Don't worry," the doctor said. "We'll get that catheter out. You're going to be OK."

"Doc, what do you think?" Dad asked.

I heard the doctor telling my parents that he believed I'd attempted suicide and asking whether they wanted me to be admitted to the psychiatric ward for evaluation. This was the normal procedure with attempted suicides.

Visions of being strapped in a bed, staring at four blank walls, washed over me. Of eating food with plastic knives and forks because the psychiatric staff wouldn't allow real utensils for us sickos to use. Of being locked in a room with no windows and no way out. A diagnosis that I was "crazy" because I had gotten drunk and swallowed a bunch of pills. No, thank you. I didn't want that.

"No." Dad shook his head. "I'm a therapist. Her mom is a social worker, and we can take care of her at home."

"Yes, we'll take care of her at home. She'll be all right." Mom took my hand. I couldn't remember a time when she had seemed so caring, so gentle.

"What about you, Karena?" the doctor asked. "You just went through a harrowing experience and could have easily died. You obviously have some issues that you're dealing with. Do you want to stay here in the hospital for evaluation or do you want to go home?"

"Yeah, I want to go home if my parents will stop fighting," I said, realizing this was a new bargaining chip for me to use.

The doctor looked at them questioningly.

"I promise you," Dad said. "We'll stop fighting."

I looked at Mom.

"Yes, Karena, I promise too. We won't fight anymore."

"OK," the doctor said. "I'll release her, but bring her back if she has any more problems."

They promised they would.

But people lie.

So Mom and Dad took me home. Mom moved back into the house so she could help take care of me. That made me happy.

For a few nights, I slept on the sofa in the living room. I would pull my knees up to my chest and wrap my arms around my shins. *If I just curl up into a ball, I won't have to face life,* I told myself. I'd be protected from everything harsh around me. But I'd still have to live with myself.

I wasn't sure why I didn't want to sleep in my room. Maybe it was because of the wild dreams I had or the red vampire eyes I saw often in my bedroom window. Maybe it was because of the weird, ghostly noises I heard from the attic as if someone were trying to claw their way out and come down the stairs that were in my closet and creep into my bedroom. Maybe I didn't want to sleep in the same room as Rachel. She had been so distant lately. Maybe the living room felt more private or safe. Maybe I felt like I could monitor the front door and watch to see if Mom was going to leave us again.

When Rachel learned about my suicide attempt, she was kinder and more respectful about my space. But she didn't trust that Mom was home for the right reasons and continued to stay away from the house most of the time. She lived in her own world and had her own circle of friends.

I stayed home from school for one week. I didn't want to face my friends or teachers, and, ironically, my parents didn't want to force me into any stressful situations. For a couple of weeks, I heard my parents arguing and crying upstairs, worried that I was going to try to kill myself again. Worried that they had caused my attempted suicide. Worried that I was forever broken. As if my wings had been clipped and I could no longer fly.

I also felt guilty and concerned that I had made things worse for my parents. That they were now fighting about what I had done and blaming themselves.

—

The wild dreams I had tormented me, and during that time, I did not sleep peacefully. I had two vivid recurring dreams. In one, I was on a train that went in a circle. And inside that circle was a big ditch—a dungeon—where people were held as prisoners. In this dream, I traveled with vampires on the train to a haunted house. Once we got there, I would either jump off the train and run to a safe area or I'd jump off on the wrong side, which was the bad side, and there, I'd be kidnapped by other vampires, their teeth dripping blood . . . and I knew it was just a matter of time before they sank their razor-sharp teeth into my neck. I had to escape. Always.

In the other dream, I would sit in a movie theater where they were playing films featuring vampires. In a film at the theater, I would become an actor—a good vampire. When I was a vampire, I could fly through the air and would often escape. I'd transform back into a human and wake up, my heart pounding in my chest.

Mom used to say that she regretted taking me to see the movie *Interview with the Vampire* and letting me watch *The Lost Boys* because she felt like they opened up my psyche to vampires, and that's why I dreamed about them. I wasn't sure that was the reason I dreamed about vampires. Maybe my dreams were simply an outlet for my fears, which helped me deal with the trauma in my life . . . or maybe the dreams added to the trauma. It's something I still wonder about.

What I did know was that these dreams were frightening and reminded me that I was always being stalked by my fears—vampires
with red eyes and long, sharp fangs.

PART FOUR

Transition

CHAPTER SEVENTEEN

White Feather at New Age People

Not sure where I'm going.
It's gotta be better than this hell is showing . . .
Wanted to reach onto my shelf,
bring death to myself . . .
Stab a blade into my wrist
and my life would be kissed.
Too much confusion . . .
Happiness, an illusion.

—Karena Dawn

Meditation.

God, I am such a loser. A failure.

Part of me was ashamed about almost killing myself. That part criticized myself for doing such a thing. If I wasn't a sinner before trying to take my own life, I believed I was now. A true full-fledged sinner. That title, in addition to my suicide attempt, led to so much shame. It would be a long time before I understood how shame can erode our courage and fuel disengagement with people. It would be a long time before I learned how to cultivate a culture of worthiness and acceptance.

And then some friends told me about meditation.

Could meditation really help me? As a teen, I didn't know much about meditation. I didn't know much about mindfulness or any of the New Age protocols to help relieve stress and pain. But after my attempted suicide, I wanted to find some answers to my problems.

I wasn't interested in going to church, but meditation was different from church, and it was different from the therapists and physicians who said they wanted to help me. Meditation was something I could do on my own, and I needed to find a safe place for my emotions—all the emotions I didn't want to feel—such as anger and sadness. Otherwise, I would cut myself again. Or take another bottle of pills.

When Megan and Emma and I went to Painted Memories Beach and wrote down our thoughts on paper and buried them beneath the big oak tree, I had thought it was the most beautiful way to "treat" my dark sadness. It gave me hope. But then I swallowed all those pills. Clearly, I needed more constructive and effective ways to address the sadness. I suggested to my friends that we go to a store in downtown Indianapolis that I'd heard about called New Age People. It was a place "for all spiritual paths," and they had psychic readings, massage therapy, and a gift shop filled with incense, books, music, crystals, aromatherapy, and yoga equipment. Every Friday evening, they held meditations.

"Meditation will help us with our problems," I explained to my girlfriends. "It's supposed to be much better than church."

Both Megan and Emma thought it sounded like a good idea. An adventure. Something fun to do.

The first Friday night that we went, we were greeted by a woman named White Feather. She was small and appeared to be in her fifties. She had long silvery hair that hung to her waist and eyes that glistened like green emeralds. There was a softness in her voice and wisdom in her lined face. "Welcome," she said. "Follow me."

White Feather ushered me and my friends into a small back room where a few people had already gathered. I could smell the incense burning along with candles. A mellow light glowed throughout the room while flute and guitar played softly in the background. Everyone was sitting on cushions on a hardwood floor. Megan, Emma, and I joined them.

"Welcome, everyone," White Feather began. "Whether this is your first time or you've been here before, I hope that this experience offers you peace of mind. Does anyone have any questions?"

Megan raised her hand. "What should we expect?"

"It's different for everyone," White Feather said. "People are so stressed in their busy lives today that sometimes meditation just helps them to wind down and relax. Meditating can help you understand the nature of your mind. And from that understanding, you learn how to calm your mind and focus your thoughts, ultimately shifting your perspective from a negative mindset to a positive one, from a place of unease to one of peace and ease."

I liked everything that White Feather had to say.

"People find us for all kinds of reasons," White Feather continued. "Some seek healing, either of the mind, body, or heart. Others come because they sense they are in some kind of life transition and they need the tools to help take the next step or make the right decision."

I definitely agreed with that. I felt like I was in some kind of transition from my sinner self to . . . just *what*, I didn't know.

"Will we change after meditation?" Emma asked.

White Feather smiled. "As you begin to quiet the world around you by focusing on your own breath, you will start to hear your inner voice—those deeper thoughts and feelings—more clearly. And, when that voice is finally heard, you will be able to tap into a stillness and a clarity that we too often crowd out with the clamor of the world and our own fears and worries. It may take a while, but it will happen."

Emma, Megan, and I grinned at each other. We didn't fully understand the "sense of stillness and clarity" part, but we knew we were in for a unique experience.

We all sat comfortably on cushions with our backs straight and our legs crossed.

"Now, dear ones, close your eyes and breathe in deeply," White Feather directed.

I inhaled slowly.

"Notice the thoughts and distractions crowding your mind," White Feather said. "Now focus on your breath; don't try and modulate it, just follow its natural rhythm. As you exhale, imagine that you are breathing out all those distracting thoughts, and as you inhale, imagine that you are breathing in all the blessings and wisdom of holy beings. Imagine these blessings take the form of a white light that clears your mind of all negative thoughts before settling in your heart."

I could hear the beating of my heart. It grew louder and louder.

"Now, join me in our chant." White Feather's voice was soft and melodious. "Om."

We repeated "om" over and over until it sounded like a chorus of beautiful harmonies.

We must have chanted for about thirty minutes when White Feather asked us to stop and enjoy the silence for a few minutes. "Silence will help you connect with your heart center, where you can hear your own inner voice speak."

A feeling of peace swept over me. It would be many years before I truly knew how to embrace the joy of meditation and apply it to my life. But at that moment, what I heard was: *It's time for you to enjoy life, Karena. You're too young to die.*

CHAPTER EIGHTEEN

Masquerade of the Wolf

The wolf . . . it stares at me.
I think it feels my pain.
Its gray coat, its blue eyes,
So pure, so innocent . . . the way it looks.
I wish I looked the same, but inside that wolf
it's probably filled with rage.
Probably wants to destroy everything in its way.
It walks with me, it guides me . . . it's always in
    front of me.
I've never seen it cry . . . why?
I don't know, I don't know.
Maybe its fears and pains are hidden inside.
I wonder if its heart aches the same as mine.
I wonder if it wants to rip its insides out, the same
    as I want.
So innocent and pure . . .
But really insecure . . .
I wonder . . .

—Karena, age thirteen

Screaming.

I was transitioning to my next state of being. Tossing out the sinner role—for I did not plan on trying to kill myself again—I was moving on. Now, I often felt like a wolf. Wild. Feral. Even after centering meditation with White Feather, I found some joy in becoming a wild, rebellious wolf. Stalking my prey. Laughing on the outside but *screaming* on the inside. Out of control.

No one could see what was going on inside. Sure, it was all a masquerade, but it was liberating and exhilarating for a time. I needed it. I was simply tired of being afraid, of being in pain. I craved some relief.

In my mind, I would be the wolf, brown eyes the color of tree bark, sinking my teeth into life and joyfully letting the blood of my prey drip from my mouth. My teeth would rip and snag through my enemies and fears, and I would be the ultimate survivor. A predator, mostly keeping her rage and pain inside but seeking out fun and wildness in any way possible.

After my time in the hospital, and after going to a few meditation sessions at New Age People, I decided I would not care about anything anymore. I was going to have fun! I locked up the pain inside my heart and threw away the key. And along with the pain, I locked away the *screams* and the *rage.* They were louder than any earthly noise. Or any heavenly noise, for that matter. But I ignored them.

In my journal, I was resolute:

> So I've decided not to die. The best thing to do is to try and hold on until I'm eighteen. I don't want people to remember me as "the girl who committed suicide." And for some reason, I don't want to let my mom down by committing such a big "sin" in her Christian mind.

—

The good news was: Mom was back home with us, for a while . . . to help me.

The bad news was: Mom was back home with us, for a while . . . to teach me more about the Antichrist and Dad's involvement in the New World Order's plot to take over the world.

The really good news was: As a wolf, I would not let Mom's delusions, or my new distrust and hatred for Dad, ruin the wild, fun times I was having in high school. I had a whole slew of new friends and some old ones: E, cocaine, weed, ketamine, uppers, downers. I would do anything but shoot heroin. I stayed away from that.

I was happy that Mom was home, but I wanted it to be normal. Instead, life was becoming more and more bizarre with each passing day.

"Don't you know that your father has been manipulating your relationships with your friends all your life?" Mom told me. "It's part of the cult. He is controlling who you see and what you do because he won't allow you to be around the wrong people who are against the cult."

I talked to Megan and Emma about my mom's conspiracy theories and the satanic cult, and they thought she was crazy. They also began to ostracize me after I tried to kill myself. They thought I was going crazy too. Without my old friends by my side, I gravitated toward groups who were into the rave scenes and the drugs that went along with them. I also hung out with the skater kids, mostly guys with long, flippy hair who dressed in baggy clothes, hoodies, and skate shoes. They toted skateboards with them whether they were riding them or not, and I thought they were sexy.

I was taller than most boys, and kids would make fun of me in school because I experimented with my hair and clothes. I went from edgy to goth, and from baggy pants and shirts to ripped blue jeans and *extra*-baggy pants. I dyed my hair pink once, and even though that would look normal in today's world, back then, it was considered odd.

By the time I was sixteen, I was going to raves all over Indiana, Kentucky, Missouri, and Ohio. They were mesmerizing, a delightful festival for the senses. The music and the lights and the crowds, all pulsing and moving, ebbing and flowing together, like one vast organism with one beating heart.

Around then, I started having random sex with guys I thought were cute. As for finding places to have sex, the boys and I were creative. We'd go to the guy's house if his parents weren't at home, or we'd go to my house if no one was there. Sometimes we'd go to the woods. Or to an alley somewhere behind a store. Anywhere. Boys were my drugs too.

—

When I first used cocaine at a high school party, I was told to start by rubbing it on my gums so that I would know it was effective by the numbing sensation. Afterward, I was taught how to snort a small line of it through a rolled dollar bill or a straw. The first sensation, of course, was discomfort in my nostril, along with some kind of substance trickling down the back of my throat. The very first "euphoric" feeling I got was from the pain of having snorted it.

On a separate occasion, I had been invited to try freebasing cocaine, and that's when I really learned how dangerously enticing it could be. The instructions were to rub some cocaine with some baking soda on a scrap of tinfoil, burn it, and inhale the smoke through a rolled tube of paper. The sensation was ultimately the same, but the faster delivery produced a stronger high and a bit more of that euphoria.

Ecstasy was one of my favorite drugs. It heightened all your senses, especially touch, everything. But it often made me sick too, and I would vomit for hours after I came down.

In order to pay for my drugs, I got part-time jobs in retail fashion stores. I also started to get into trouble with the police. Once, I was arrested and put in jail for doing drugs, and another time for stealing NoDoz caffeine pills. I was even held for stealing lotion from Bath & Body Works at the mall. And along with my school friends, we were busted for underage drinking.

It became a regular thing for the cops to raid the houses where we were partying. We'd run out the back and try to hide in the trees and bushes. The cops always found us, though, and loaded us into their vans to take us to the station. At first, we would laugh, thinking it was funny. But as the high wore off, we all became irritable and furious.

Dad always came and got me out of jail, but instead of being grateful, I'd just be mad at him and do the same thing the next day.

—

There were also some good times that didn't involve raves and drugs or sex, times when Mom was around and in a normal mood. But even those times could prove damaging. She took me to Chicago to meet with modeling agencies. She thought I'd be successful because I was so tall and skinny, but like many high school girls, I was very insecure about my looks. I loved looking at magazines like *Seventeen*, and I dreamed about being on the cover one day. I would try to dress like those cover girls and style my hair in the same way.

I quickly signed with an agency. They wanted to send me to Europe to model high-end fashion, but for that, I had to lose ten pounds. I didn't ever think I had a weight problem before. I was already thin, but I knew how strict the modeling agencies were. As a result, I developed bulimia, an eating disorder where I would force myself to vomit after eating. Many of my girlfriends did this. It almost became a sick competition on who could be the thinnest.

Fortunately, Mom was so inconsistent with her on-again, off-again mothering that she let the modeling go. After a couple of years, I recovered from my eating disorder.

—

Dad was distant from us when he was home. Mom would pop in and stay awhile, then she'd leave for days at a time. When she did reappear, it was generally because she thought she could "save" us from Satan and the apocalypse, which she believed was going to take place in the near future.

Mom kept her apartment during this time, and whenever she decided to leave, she would try to entice me and Rachel to come and stay with her. I wouldn't go. And neither would Rachel.

Even though I told myself that I was a wolf and that I was having the time of my life at all the raves and with the drugs, I was still very insecure. I still felt abandoned.

This pain was hidden from the world. But I knew it was still there. Deep, deep inside. Like a wolf who traveled the wilds looking for food in a wintry land that is barren and frozen, I was starving for sustenance.

PART FIVE

Homeless

CHAPTER NINETEEN

Turkey Run State Park

"Homeless"
Poem by Rachel Sahaidachny

She chose to live
On wildflowers and clover
She chose to drink
Mud collected in ditches
Some might question my choice to use
The word "chose"
She chose not to take her injections
She chose to live on the road
Her eyes so blue
Everything she sees or doesn't drowns
It's possible I will never see her
She always moves farther away
While she wanders, I wait
For news of her death
Hope she might dissolve
Unnoticed except for the bit of her
I can't spit out
Biting the thick of my tongue
Red split in the white coating

I choke every morning
My head says quit

Dirty hair, dirty fingers.

Even though I was suspicious of Dad and wondered if he really was part of an international cult, I still knew that he was trying to keep our family and home life together. I knew he was trying to keep our home life "normal" the best he could when Mom disappeared and then reappeared. But, of course, how could anyone expect this to be normal?

Kids need their moms, but as teenagers, Rachel and I *especially* needed her. We needed the consistency of Mom and Dad being at home with us. Of dinner together. Of grocery shopping together. Of watching movies on Friday nights at home together. There was no consistency at all.

Each day when Dad came home from work, and I was there, he'd bounce through the doorway and look expectantly at the stairs as if he thought Mom might come down any moment. I noticed the sadness in his eyes when he was greeted by nothing more than an empty stairwell.

For the months after my suicide attempt, Mom kept her apartment in Indianapolis and worked as a maid, coming home sporadically and acting as though she'd never been away. But the times away from home began stretching longer and longer until it had been six weeks since anyone had heard from her.

One evening, Dad, Rachel, and I drove over to Mom's apartment hoping to find her, but no one was there. Her closets had been cleaned out, and there were no personal items anywhere. Old food wrappers from fast-food restaurants were piled high in the garbage can. Apparently, this time, Mom had abandoned her apartment as well. We had no idea where she was.

I panicked silently.

Dad kept saying, "Girls, she'll turn up. She always does."

I wanted to believe Dad, but none of us knew how sick she really was. Not this time. I felt that old sense of dread overcome me. In fact, *dread* became its own entity, pushing against me like an invisible gate. Trying to smother me with fear.

I breathed in deeply and tried to pretend everything was OK.

Sadness had also become my albatross. My music, the raves, the sex and drugs, my escapes. But the sadness . . . it stayed with me. Deep within, it lay like dirty snow over every other emotion, the dread, the fear, graying my spirit, tainting all that could bring me joy and relief.

Then one evening, out of the blue, Mom called our house. Dad answered the phone and held the receiver out so Rachel and I could hear the conversation.

"Where the hell are you?" Dad asked her.

"Don't yell at me, Nick," Mom said, her voice defiant and willful. "I'm fine."

"I want to see you. The girls want to see you." Dad glanced at me and Rachel. There was panic in his voice.

"OK. I guess we could meet."

"Where are you?" Dad pressed again.

Silence.

"Please," Dad said. "Tell me where you are so the girls and I can meet you."

Finally, Mom gave Dad directions to where she was.

When Dad hung up, he said, "C'mon, girls, we're going to see your mom. She's at Turkey Run State Park."

"Tonight?" I swallowed hard.

"Yes, tonight."

I had heard of Turkey Run State Park but had never been there. Dad said it was in Marshall, Indiana, an hour and a half from Indianapolis.

"I'm not sure if she's been camping out there or what," Dad said as he rummaged through the kitchen drawers, looking for a map. "I didn't ask too many questions."

"But she's all right?" I asked. I bit my lower lip out of nervousness.

"I think so," Dad said. "They have bathroom facilities there . . . things like that, if she's camping out. It's not as if she's in a secluded forest somewhere where there are no people."

Rachel raised her eyebrows as if she wasn't sure she believed Dad.

I just wanted to feel that all would be OK.

"C'mon," Dad said, grabbing the Indiana map, folding it, and stuffing it in his jeans pocket. "Your mom said she'd be there, waiting for us. Let's go."

We grabbed our jackets, a couple of water bottles, and headed out the door.

Dad, Rachel, and I said very little on the way. All of us were hopeful. And all of us were afraid our hopes would be squashed.

The evening sky was deepening and quickly turning to nighttime, stars and the crescent moon shining overhead. I had no idea what we would find once we got there.

"Are there bears in the park?" I asked.

"Bears? No, I don't think so," Dad said. "Probably a lot of turkeys, deer, and beavers around Sugar Creek. But I think your mom is safe there. It's a popular tourist area, and there's even an inn there, thank God."

"Oh." I turned my attention to the car window, still hopeful but cautious.

Rachel barely spoke at all.

Each minute seemed to stretch into an hour, as if we would never get there. But, finally, we did.

As we entered the park grounds, a big sign welcomed us.

I breathed a sigh of relief. We were there. Mom would be there. *She promised she'd be there.* We just had to find where she was parked.

We drove around for a few minutes, straining our eyes as we scrutinized the cars parked around the grounds. Even though it was getting dark, I could see that Turkey Run State Park was beautiful, with deep canyons tucked beneath sandstone cliffs and serene groves of beech, sycamore, and hemlock. Dad said there were numerous rugged trails throughout the park.

"Where is she?" asked Rachel, sounding impatient.

"Look!" Dad said. We saw an overhead light over a garbage bin. A pay phone was nearby. That was the phone she probably used to call us. Mom's car was parked there too.

"There! There she is!" I shouted, pointing at the car.

"Is that her in the car?" Rachel asked.

"I think so," Dad said.

I saw a small figure hunched over in the driver's seat. *Is it Mom? Is she OK?*

Dad pulled up close to the garbage bin and parked the car, then Rachel and I got out and walked over to where Mom sat.

Oh . . . my . . . God! Shit, shit, shit. I shouldn't have been surprised to see her like this, but I was.

"Linda, open up," Dad said, tapping on the window.

She looked up at us and blinked her eyes, as if trying to recognize us. Then she slowly opened the car door and got out. Her fingernails were ragged and torn as if she had been chewing on them. Her hands were covered in black grime. She had lost so much weight, her jeans were now baggy, and her blue mohair sweater was stretched out and full of holes as if she had stretched it a thousand ways. Her boots were scuffed and caked with mud. It was almost as if someone had stolen her original clothes and she had rummaged through garbage bins to find something else to wear.

Good God! Where has she been? What has she been doing?

"Mom!" I shouted.

I wanted to reach out and grab her, but I held back. A part of me was afraid to touch her. I think we were all a little bit afraid.

Mom's beautiful, bright blue eyes, usually so full of warmth, had frozen over all gray and icy. She felt far away. *Away from Dad. Away from me and Rachel.* I wanted to tell her it wasn't hopeless, that we loved her like always and she would be safe with us, but she probably wouldn't believe me. I wanted to rekindle her warmth, but her insides seemed too damp and cold. I always thought Mom had pain inside, but now it was visible on her face and body. I wished it would go away. Didn't she see us hurting too?

"Hello, Karena, Nick . . . Rachel." Again, she blinked her eyes as if she were coming out of a trance. Her voice was monotone as if we had just seen each other earlier that day. Not six weeks ago.

Rachel stood back behind me and kept her distance.

"Linda, c'mon, honey, let's all sit together on a bench somewhere and talk awhile." I knew that Dad didn't want to spook her. If any of us said too much, she might drive off and leave us.

Silence.

"Can we visit awhile and talk?" Dad asked as gently as he could.

"Please, Mom?" I begged. I bit my lower lip hard, trying not to cry.

"Let's go up by the lodge." Her voice was low, raspy, and hoarse. "There's some benches up there."

"Sure," Dad said. It wasn't far from where we were.

Mom was frail, not much more than skin and bones. A skeleton. Her brown hair hung like a dirty, stringy mop around her face. Lines crinkled around her blue eyes that were now dull and faded gray. The brightness was gone. Her face was smudged with dirt and dried blood. Or was that ketchup? *What had she done to herself?* It looked as if she had been rummaging with her face in the garbage bin.

It was embarrassing to see Mom like this, and we couldn't help but notice that there were nicely dressed tourists going in and out of the lodge. They glanced at us as they passed and quickly looked away. As if we were all homeless people. They didn't want to be associated with us.

Mom was a shadow of the mother I knew just a few weeks ago. Gaunt. Emaciated. Ghostly.

It suddenly dawned on me: She didn't just arrange to meet us at the park. This was where she had been living! In her car!

I was appalled. Even Rachel had watery eyes. It was all I could do to keep from bursting into tears.

Dad seemed determined not to break down.

Mom is homeless! It didn't sound logical that my mom would be a homeless person. *How can I explain that to my friends? To anyone?*

After we sat on the park benches, Dad asked, "Linda, have you been living all alone in your car?"

"No," she said.

"Has somebody been with you?" We all glanced around the park. None of us saw any signs of anyone else "living" there.

"I have a friend." Linda folded her arms, almost defiantly.

"Who's your friend, Mom?" I asked, a little too hopeful.

"Barney," she said. "His name is Barney."

"Linda, who's Barney?" Dad asked softly.

"A cute little brown mouse." Her eyes were glazed over as if she were trying to remember.

"A mouse? Mom! A mouse isn't your friend!" I shouted.

Rachel rolled her eyes. "She's making that up."

"No, really," Mom said. "A little mouse I named Barney has been my friend. I've shared my food with him. He's kept me good company."

"Where did you get your food, Linda?" Dad asked.

"Here and there."

"Where?" he pressed.

"People throw out good food in the garbage bins. Sandwiches that have never been taken out of their wrappers. I didn't want it to go to waste."

"Oh, for heaven's sake," Rachel said while standing, her hands on her hips.

Dad threw her a look.

"Is that all that you've eaten?" Dad asked.

"Snow." Linda started mumbling. "Snowwww."

"Snow? You ate snow?" Dad asked.

"It's all right to eat snow," she said. "When I was little, Mom made snow cream all the time. Just like ice cream but made out of snow."

"It hasn't snowed for three weeks," Dad said.

"I ate snow then," she said.

"Look, Linda, come home with us," Dad said. "The girls really want you to come home. You can have the bedroom, and I'll sleep on the couch. It's warm there, and we have plenty of food."

"Look, I'm fine," she said. "I need my space. I only called because I wanted you to know I'm OK."

"Please, Linda," Dad persisted. "You do not need to be out here. The weather is still cold. You have a nice home. Come back with us."

"Mom, please come home," I said.

Rachel said nothing. I don't think she wanted Mom to come back with us.

"There is one thing I need," Mom said.

"What's that?" Dad asked.

"I need some gas. The park manager told me I had to move my car, and I'm running on empty . . . and I don't have any extra money for gas."

"OK," Dad said.

So that is the reason she wanted us to come, I thought. *She doesn't care about seeing us at all. She just wants money for gas!*

Dad told us to stay with Mom while he drove to the nearest gas station and filled up a container with gas.

"OK," Rachel and I said. I didn't really want to be left alone with Mom. I was still kind of scared of her.

"I won't be long," Dad said.

Rachel and I sat with Mom on the park bench without talking. There were no words to say. Mom didn't love us enough to come home. She preferred the company of a mouse named Barney and an old car to live in. I couldn't even begin to put into words the heartbreaking reality of the moment.

True to his word, Dad wasn't gone long. He brought the gasoline back to Mom's car and filled it up.

Dad asked her one last time, "Linda, will you please follow us home?"

"I need my space," she said. "I have places I can go . . . friends who will help me."

Of course we didn't believe her.

By now, even Rachel begged Mom to come home with us.

"I'll be all right," she said. "I'll let you know where I am. And there are shelters I can go to if I need to. I just need to be alone for a while. Don't worry about me. I'll call, I promise."

We finally relented. Dad gave her all the cash he had. Probably about fifty bucks, and we left her sitting in her car, hunched over the steering wheel, supposedly with her friend Barney. The mouse.

On the drive home, we were all sobbing. Even Rachel. Our sobs were so loud, they drowned out the sound of the car's engine.

We would never be the same again.

We were in mourning.

—

Dear Mom,

I feel so raw today, uncovered and exposed.

There was hope . . . before today. Just a tiny flicker against the wind. I was so naive thinking everything would be all right. I wanted to shout to you, Mom. In that moment, when you saw us, you had a choice for

*kindness or cruelty. It took no time for you to decide.
You saw us, looking at you so hopeful. How is it that you
could see us suffering and choose to make it all worse?*

*Dad tried his best. He really did. Rachel and I tried
our best to get you to come home too. But you didn't
care. You simply DID. NOT. CARE.*

*I feel ragged and breathless. I silently cry out to you,
"Mom, I love you. Please come back to us. Come sit with
me and eat pizza. Call me your little girl again. Let's
work out to your favorite workout videos. Please don't
abandon us. Look at me, Mom, because I am falling,
and if I keep falling into the void, I am afraid I'll never
get out."*

—

Mom hadn't even hugged us, and I'd been afraid to hug her. Afraid I
would crush her. Or get blood or grime on my clothes. I needed her. I
needed her love. But she was gone. So the only way to escape this pain
was to say, "What the fuck?" I could not let myself think about it.

CHAPTER TWENTY

White Tiger

Walk with me
Talk with me
Guide me through time
Save me from only he
Who made me drink wine
Hate them all
Kill them all
Watch them die
They did it all
I can't cry
When I see them fall

—Karena, age thirteen

Hollowness.

Many of us are running away from the hollowness of disappointment and abandonment. The courage it takes to face this emotional vacuum is tremendous, and I continually work on it. This "work" is never-ending.

I have a difficult time remembering whether I was loved as a child. When I look back at photographs of my childhood, it *looks* like I was loved. I must have been. My arms wrapped around Mom. Her arms wrapped around me. She's so pretty. Her dark hair clean and shining. Her teeth brilliantly white. And she's laughing. I'm laughing. Our relatives are laughing. Sharing the silliest of moments. Sharing real family time.

What I am learning is that as the hardened crust of our outer being cracks open, as the walls of inner separation break down along with the many layers of subterfuge, there is a light that shines through, just like the great musician Leonard Cohen said. That inner light of spirit is always there.

That inner light surrounds a fire that burns deeply in the heart. With each unfolding of self, we witness another layer of consciousness rise to the surface. The soul begins to unveil itself and manifest more profoundly, supporting body, mind, and life.

But it took me a long while before I realized all of that. As a teen, I didn't possess that kind of awareness.

—

Yesterday was a nightmare day. Rachel and I went with Dad to visit Mom at Turkey Run State Park, almost two hours from our home. She looked like a mouse. Skinny. And homeless. I think she's dying. And that's really all I want to say about that right now.

My birthday is in a few days. It's gonna be very odd because it will be the first one without my mom. But hey, that's OK. Sure, my dad will try to make it special, but he's clueless about what's really going on with me. He'll say things like, "How are you? You doin' OK?" He's such an act. Dad's always tryin' to get us to tell him what we're thinking, but Rachel and I have to hide our thoughts.

I'll be fourteen years old in a few days. But who really cares? There's still four years before I can legally move out. All I really want to do is smoke some weed or cigarettes, maybe take some LSD, and hang out at Painted Memories Beach with my friends. Just

the other day we went swimming in the muddy water.
We'll probably get some disease or worms because the
water is so dirty. We took lots of pictures, and I'll pick
them up at Walgreens today. And there's a party this
weekend and I'm going to have a grand time. I'd like
to go to New Age People before then. I'm really liking
the meditation sessions. Don't know if they help me or
not, but I like them. They're so cool. OK. Gotta go. Bye
for now.

—

All white tigers have blue eyes. Beautiful, stunning bright-blue eyes. I didn't realize that until my experience at New Age People.

After Nightmare Day at Turkey Run State Park, I needed solace, peace, and calm. On the outside, I was my usual "girl who likes to party and have fun," but on the inside, I was screaming. I hated Mom, and I hated Dad. I hated almost everyone. And even though I wanted to transition and have a better attitude and life, the call of the wild beckoned daily.

Even though I hadn't been hanging out with Megan and Emma much anymore, I called them every now and then. That week, I insisted that we go to New Age People on Friday night. They said sure. They knew that afterward we'd find some boys and do drugs. It was all we thought about. Mostly.

But NAP was becoming a different kind of fun for us. Almost like a drug itself, the meditations were starting to open us to something *beyond* ourselves. As if there were different levels of our "selves" that unfolded each time we meditated.

Like always, we were greeted by White Feather. She knew us quite well by then. As usual, we went into the small back room where other "seekers" were gathered. That's what White Feather called us: "seekers." People who were seeking spiritual enlightenment and self-awareness.

The incense greeted us, along with the scent of burning candles. Flute music played through the speakers. My friends and I took off our shoes and sat down on the cushions.

"Welcome, dear ones," White Feather said. "I see that everyone present has been here several times, but does anyone have any questions?" She usually began like this.

"I know we always chant 'om,'" said Megan, "but are there other words for chanting?"

"If you have a sacred name or spiritual guide in your life, you can chant that name, or Vedic mantras during meditation," said White Feather. "Some Christians chant 'Jesus.' The Sufis chant 'Hu,' which is an ancient name for God. 'Om' is one of the most widely used mantras by Buddhists in meditation and in the world, and that's why we chant it here. But it's up to you."

I was restless and wanted to get started. I didn't care what word we used to chant.

We closed our eyes and began our chant of "om." I was aware of the strong drumming sound of my heart beating, which seemed to blend in with the sound of chanting. Usually, I experienced a peaceful calm settling over my body. This time was different.

In my soul-body, I traveled to another place and time. White Feather had explained to us many times that when we had out-of-body experiences, it was our soul-body traveling beyond our physical body to other worlds.

—

I opened my eyes in my soul-body. I was no longer in the back room of NAP. I could not hear "om" anymore. I could not see my friends. I was alone in a barren wilderness of snow and ice.

Icicles dangled from shadowy skeletons of trees. There was a river, frozen solid, covered with ice so thick it showed reflections as clear as a mirror of the gray sky and trees that flanked either side. I thought briefly of Painted Memories Beach—the place that held so many of my secrets and dreams—but I knew this place, this "other world," was different.

Ice was everywhere. Cold, wet, slippery as glass. A bitter wind sliced through the air, whispering secrets, but I couldn't hear what it was saying. I felt as though I was heading to an out-of-control place, dangerous, deadly, lethal, treacherous. *What was the wind saying?*

Icicles, glistening and dripping from dark tree limbs like winter's daggers . . . ice crystals sparkling on the tops of trees, beautiful, white, gleaming.

Where was this place?

I thought briefly about my home. In the winter, our Tudor house often reminded me of an ice palace when it snowed. The icicles on the porch were bigger than dragon teeth, and the roof would sparkle white under a blanket of freezing crystals. And our driveway became a deathly sheet of black ice. Even the windows of our house would frost over with intricate snowflake patterns. It was frigid and beautiful, brutal and untamed. A metaphor for my teenage life.

I breathed in deeply . . . *waiting* . . . for what, I didn't know.

Then something magical happened. There were white tigers all around me. Maybe five or six, or more. They stepped out from behind the trees in the forest and walked toward me. I think I half expected snarls or growls, a flash of teeth. I half expected them to attack me. But they didn't.

One came closer. Like the others, she was as white as snow with brown stripes all over her body. Magnificent. The most beautiful creature I'd ever seen. Her stance was confident and her body muscular. Her steps were fluid and she moved without apparent effort.

I stood transfixed, unable to move as the white tiger walked up to me and looked me in the eye. I was greeted by hazy, faded blue eyes. *My mother's eyes.* Full of pain, confusion, and loss.

I began to cry, and in a flash, my mother's eyes were gone and in their place were the tiger's eyes. Clear crystal-blue eyes that shone with wisdom and clarity.

White Tiger began to speak to me. I couldn't remember everything she said, but I did remember this: "You have to leave, Karena. You can't stay here in this city."

"Why?" I asked White Tiger.

"You're drowning here," White Tiger said.

"But I'm too young to leave legally," I said.

"Time will pass quickly. You must remember to leave when the time is right. You will not survive to become your best if you stay here."

Chills ran down my spine.

"Do not give up, Karena," White Tiger said. "You have many great things to accomplish in this life."

Did she really just say that? Or is this my imagination?

"Remember you are loved, Karena," White Tiger added. "People are waiting to meet you. To love you. Now you must run."

"Run?"

"Just run."

So I turned and ran across the snow and ice, not looking back. White Tiger was chasing me away from the other tigers, urging me to run as fast as I could. I wasn't sure if it was because I was in danger or what.

A dense dark-green forest appeared before me. It looked ancient. The trees looked as if they had lived thousands of years. I strained to hear birdsong and animals that surely roamed the forest. The trees danced in the wind, and the wind became music, and there was the sound of running water in a stream somewhere. The drone of insects hummed, while little frogs croaked as they searched for food. A brilliant white shaft of light illuminated a path before me. *Where will it take me?*

There was no ice and snow in this forest. It looked welcoming and peaceful. As I was standing with the ancient forest before me and the icy arctic land behind me, I turned to ask White Tiger why I had to leave.

"You're dying here, Karena," White Tiger said. "You can't stay."

I stepped forward in the direction of the forest when a clear large bubble floated in front of me and picked me up. I rode inside this bubble over the forest and up into the sky. It was an endless canvas where the colors segued from blue to salmon, bright pink to orange. We passed low-hanging clouds that gave me the impression they were filled with wonder and possibilities. And even far above me, I could see the night sky speckled with stars and the glowing moon. I knew the sky was alive, growing in each passing moment, constantly changing for the world to see.

—

"Om" was the next sound I heard. I opened my eyes, and there I sat with my friends Megan and Emma, White Feather, and everyone else.

I couldn't move for a few minutes. The experience had been powerful. Beautiful. Prophetic.

After that, I often wondered if the forest was a better place for me. It had to be. White Tiger was showing me that there was a forest full of opportunities waiting for me when the time was right. And that time would come.

There was no doubt about it. I had to leave Indiana.

When I was old enough. When the time was right.

CHAPTER TWENTY-ONE

Painted Feelings

Painting is a reflection of who we are.

—Karena Dawn

I am an artist.

At school, I tried to pretend like everything was OK. But nothing was OK. My best friends, Megan and Emma, whom I had spent so many days with at the river of PMB and meditating with White Feather at NAP, were drifting away. They would hang out with me if I wanted to meditate, but if I wanted to simply party, they were too busy. Mom's actions and my actions put distance between us. In fact, I felt like a stigma followed me everywhere. When I walked down the hallways at school, I noticed groups of students whispering with each other when they saw me. I was sure they were talking about Mom. About me.

One day, I looked for Natalie, one of my new drug buddies. She had long blonde hair, the color of corn silk, and always wore skinny jeans and black hoodies. Natalie had a way of attracting the boys. She put on a tough-girl act, but I knew it was a facade to mask her vulnerability. I saw through her charade. No one else did. No one saw the real her. Just like nobody saw the real me.

I couldn't find her before art class.

It was the last class of the day. On Friday. Art class.

"Paint your feelings today," said Mrs. Klink, the art teacher.

My feelings? Immediately, I thought of sadness and abandonment and dark shadows. Shadows that haunted me night and day with hopes that Mom would return home. I also felt defiance that said, "I don't give a big fuck." And red vampire eyes. Rebellious eyes. Those demon eyes that still stared at me through my bedroom window at night.

Then I thought about meditation sessions with White Feather and white light. And the wolf. I thought of myself as the wolf. Hunting my prey. The boys. The sex. The drugs.

I grabbed my paintbrush and started frantically swirling colors on the canvas propped on the easel in front of me. A blur of shades representing pain, demons, and shadows. And in one corner, a burst of white light trying to edge its way into my life. I began painting an abstract of a ghastly figure. A woman in a white gown with green skin. She looked like an alien of sorts. It was Mom.

The bell rang, snapping me out of my concentration.

Someone leaned over me.

I jumped.

"Sorry!" said Mrs. Klink. "I didn't mean to startle you. Do you mind if I take a look?"

"Of course not," I said.

The teacher sat down beside me, studying my painting. I wanted to get out of there. I wanted to find Natalie so we could drive to a rave together later.

Mrs. Klink didn't say anything for a few moments. *Did she like it?*

"This is very powerful, Karena," she said. "The emotion, the depth—it truly affects the viewer—it affects *me*."

"I've heard that before," I said nonchalantly.

"That's a good thing, Karena. You can affect the viewer and make them feel something that's deep."

I just stared at her. If she wanted to talk deep, I could talk deep. But right now, all I wanted was to find a blunt or do some meth or cocaine—anything to get high—I just wanted to escape.

"Is everything OK at home, Karena?" She had a disturbed look on her face. No doubt she had heard the stories about my crazy mom who ran away from us all the time.

"Everything's fine!" I said quickly, my voice a little too bright, a little too forced.

Mrs. Klink leaned forward. "I don't think you know how extraordinary you are, Karena. I have worked with several gifted students before, but you're by far the most talented I've ever known. You paint with vision. And that's unique."

"Really?" *Did she truly believe in my art?*

"Yes, really. I hope you'll stay true to your vision as you grow in your life."

"Thank you, Mrs. Klink. I'll remember what you said today."

I heard the kids whispering and talking as they streamed past me to exit the classroom. Probably joking about my paintings. Probably making fun of me.

I ignored them.

"Have a good weekend, Karena, and I'll see you Monday," said Mrs. Klink.

I gathered my pens and put them in my backpack. I put the brushes in a jar of linseed oil and left the classroom.

An electric charge ran through me. It was excitement and energy. A feeling of affirmation but self-doubt too. *Does Mrs. Klink really think I'm talented?*

Nah, she probably says that to everyone.

I ran down the hallway and to the back entrance, where the school buses and cars were parked. Natalie was in the alleyway.

"I've been looking for you," I said.

Natalie lit a cigarette and took a drag. Then she handed it to me. I put it to my lips and inhaled.

"How was art class?" Natalie asked.

"Mrs. Klink said I was talented."

"Nice to get a teacher to compliment you," Natalie said.

"Uh-huh. My mom's an artist too."

"So you must be really talented with your mom being an artist too," Natalie said, grabbing the cigarette from me and taking a long drag.

I shrugged. I didn't feel like talking about Mom. In fact, I seldom talked about Mom with anyone anymore because I didn't want to lose friends.

Natalie crushed the cigarette out on the bottom of her shoe. "Hey, you wanna still go to the rave tonight?"

"Absolutely," I said.

"Well, let's go to my house first and get high," Natalie said. "I've got meth and some E, and my parents won't be home because they go for drinks after work on Fridays."

"Sounds good," I said. "We'll be ready for the rave!"

I felt excited as we left the school grounds—and not just about the rave. But because someone recognized that I was an artist.

CHAPTER TWENTY-TWO

Broken Love Pieces, Broken Heart Pieces

"Face of Love"
Song and lyrics by Nick Ivanovich

The sun rises and the sun sets
Like any other day.
Sometimes the sadness in my heart
Just won't go away.
Redeem my heart.
Be the torch in the dark.
The ways of this world remain the same
But in that desperate hour of the day.
There's a glimpse of glory in the face of love.
There is so much beauty in the face of love.
And I can see a bit of heaven in the face of love.

Love pieces . . .
 *She sat motionless, unaware of the time that had
passed . . . just staring into the abyss. Her eyes fixated
on nothing at all. She appeared to have no thoughts. No
spirit. No soul. Perhaps she knew her fate was sealed.
Perhaps she was already gone from this world.*

Heart pieces . . .

    Mom, I could write you a thousand letters, each one the same as the last. I miss you and I want you here with me. With us. My beautiful mother with your bright blue eyes and your warm smile and your tormented soul. Without you, I feel like a vital part of me is missing. Like a broken toy or a machine that doesn't work right anymore. Like my heart is broken into a hundred little pieces. Little heart pieces . . . Can I ever let go of the hope that we will be a family again?

—

I continued going to raves with Natalie and my other party friends. And I kept painting my feelings in art class. I took pride in the fact that Mrs. Klink had called me an artist.

One night, Mom called Dad. It had only been a few weeks after we'd seen her at Turkey Run State Park. Mom told him that she was in a women's shelter in Terre Haute, Indiana.

When Dad told me and Rachel where she was, I asked if we could go get her.

Dad said, "Look, they're providing shelter and nourishment for her, so we don't have to worry about her. She probably wouldn't come with us even if we tried."

"Is she coming back?" I asked.

"I don't know," said Dad.

"I don't know how you can stay married to her," Rachel said. "She hasn't been your wife for years."

I threw Rachel a sharp look. We had no idea what Dad was going through.

Dad didn't say anything.

Well after I was out on my own, Dad told me that, at the time, he'd hired an attorney to help him because he was emotionally exhausted and didn't know what his legal rights were. He stayed in the situation with Mom much longer than many people would.

Soon after calling us, Mom left the shelter and moved into an apartment in Terre Haute. One day, her landlord called Dad. "Are you Nick Ivanovich, the guy who's married to Linda?"

"Yes, is something wrong?" Dad asked.

"I'm not sure. I found a note on the windshield of her car. It's been there for days. It was a note to you and gave your phone number."

"What does she want?" Dad asked.

"She wants to meet you in a park in southern Illinois. Linda said she'd be waiting there for you."

"Do you know where this place is?" Dad asked.

"It's fifty miles away from Terre Haute. I can give you directions."

"Do you know how she got there if she didn't take her car?"

"I guess she walked, got a ride, or hitchhiked, and left her car right here in our parking lot. Probably out of gas or something. She's been acting a little strange, to tell you the truth."

Dad immediately called the crisis hotline in that region and asked them if they could help find Mom. When he'd hung up, Dad turned to me and Rachel. "Girls, we'll need to go pick up Mom once they find her."

"No," said Rachel. "I'm not coming. I don't want to go through that again. Not now. Not ever."

"What about you, Karena?"

"Don't go, Karena," Rachel said. "Mom just wants to play on your sympathy."

I was torn. "But, Rachel," I said, "Mom needs us."

"It's up to you," Dad said. "Maybe your grandmother Rose will come."

Dad called Grammy and explained what was happening. She said she would go with him.

We sat in the kitchen waiting for a phone call. Finally, it rang. It was a police officer saying that they'd found Mom. "She's sitting on a bench in a park in Illinois, outside Terre Haute."

"Is she OK?" Dad asked.

"Yeah, seems fine," the police officer said. "We approached her, and she said she was waiting for her husband."

"Can you take her to the police station and keep her there until I get there?" Dad knew Mom would be safe in a police station.

"We don't have enough evidence that she's a danger to herself," the police officer said. "And we can't just take her in because she's sitting on a park bench."

"Look, she's in a psychotic state," Dad said. "I've been through this before."

"Sir, she has a right to be sitting on the park bench," the police officer said. "She's not hurting anyone, and she's not hurting herself. There's nothing more we can do."

Dad hung up and called Mom's landlord again. "They found her at a park, but the police officer won't take her in because she's not causing any disturbance. Can you give me directions to this park?"

"Sure," the landlord said. "You going to pick her up?"

"Yeah," Dad said. "I'm bringing Linda's mom. Look, Thomas, would you mind going with us? We can come by and pick you up at the apartment complex."

"Sure," he said. "I'm happy to help."

"Thanks."

By now, I had decided I'd go with Dad and Grammy. I thought perhaps she'd come home with us if she saw me. Rachel could stay behind, but I would go. I wasn't ready to give up on Mom completely.

Dad seemed relieved.

As we drove toward Terre Haute, we didn't say much. Here I was, once again, riding in a car to find my homeless mother. I was sad but angry too. I noticed that Grammy kept wiping her eyes and blowing her nose. I knew she was crying softly.

Finally, Dad found the apartment complex and picked up Thomas. He seemed like a nice man. A big, burly guy who could have been anyone's grandfather. Grammy and I sat in the back seat while Thomas rode up front with Dad.

Surreally, we made everyday chitchat about the weather while driving.

None of us wanted to talk about a woman who had abandoned her children and husband, and then her apartment and car, and somehow made it fifty miles away from where she was staying. None of us wanted to talk about psychosis and the true meaning of Mom's actions.

By the time we got to the park, it was ten p.m. and the night was chilled with a blustery wind. It felt like we were characters in an Alfred Hitchcock movie as Dad wove through the trees on the pitch-dark, winding country roads. Through the car window, I couldn't find the moon or any stars.

Then a coyote darted across the street; it was grungy, scary looking. I screamed as Dad swerved to avoid hitting it. We were absolutely in the middle of nowhere.

But. *Finally.* We saw her. On the bench next to a picnic table.

Grammy let out a cry and grabbed my hand.

Dad and Thomas threw each other a quick look and clenched their jaws.

A wave of nausea overcame me. I wanted to vomit.

I broke into a thousand heart pieces. Right then and there.

I was sure that Dad's and Grammy's hearts had broken too. Into a thousand love pieces. A thousand heart pieces.

Dad was broken.

Grammy was broken.

I was broken too.

In many ways, it felt like a rerun of the scene at Turkey Run State Park. Only, this time, Mom wasn't in her car. She had nothing with her but the clothes on her back. Not even the little friendly mouse, Barney.

Dad and Thomas got out of the car and approached Mom. In the back seat, Grammy held my hand as she rolled down the car window. We were close enough that we could hear their conversation. There was a pole nearby with a light, but it wasn't very bright.

"Linda, are you OK?" Dad asked. His voice was small and quiet. "I brought Thomas with us. He knew where the park was."

"Linda, what do you need?" asked Thomas. "Can I help?"

Mom sat crumpled on the bench, folded over the picnic table, a tattered mess of ripped clothes and muck. An almost skeletal frame. I'd never seen her cheekbones jutting out like that before. And a greasy brown mane surrounded her face, covering her eyes. A dirty polyurethane cup sat on the table in front of her. It was as if she was breathing without really being alive.

She barely looked up when Dad and Thomas spoke.

"Nick, we have to go on a mission," she mumbled.

Dad and Thomas threw each other a quick look.

"Honey, we can talk about a mission later."

She didn't respond.

"C'mon, Linda." He was trying to be as gentle as possible.

Then Dad put his arms around Mom and scooped her up like she was a rag doll.

"Put me down, Nick." Her voice was weak and barely audible, and she didn't fight him.

Dad carried her to the car. Grammy and I moved over so he could put her in the back with us. The stench of rot was strong. Mom was filthy and smelled like garbage and sewage, and her eyes were glassy and strange.

Grammy held her like she was a baby while we both cried.

Mom continued to mumble, "Nick, we have a mission . . . must get away from the devil . . . the cabal . . ."

No one said a word. We let Mom ramble on and on.

Dad drove to the psychiatric hospital in Terre Haute. It was midnight when we arrived.

We all followed Dad as he carried Mom into the hospital.

"What's wrong with her?" asked the admitting clerk. I couldn't detect any kindness whatsoever in the clerk's face.

"She's been homeless," said Dad.

"This is the wrong place for her," the clerk said.

"No, really, she needs a bed, and a doctor should see her," Dad insisted. "I'm a therapist, and I know you can do a seventy-two-hour psychiatric hold. She has a mental disorder."

Finally, he convinced the clerk, and they put Mom in a wheelchair and whisked her off down the hallway. She didn't even look back at us.

"I'm so sorry about all of this," Thomas said. "She could be so nice at times, and then act so weird and strange at other times."

"I know," Dad said. "We've been dealing with that as a family for a long time. Thanks for calling me. She could have died out there in that park."

"Glad to help."

"Is it all right if I leave her car in your parking lot? I'll arrange to have a tow truck pick it up, if that's OK with you."

"Sure," said Thomas. "Whatever you need."

After the psychiatric hold, the doctors transferred Mom to Methodist Hospital in Indianapolis. She was there for three weeks and was diagnosed as having paranoid schizophrenia—the same as her father. She'd received this diagnosis before, but I was only now under-standing what it really meant.

I didn't like the fact that this was inherited from family members.

Did that mean I would inherit this mental disease?

Would I become crazy like my mother?

This thought chilled me to the bone.

CHAPTER TWENTY-THREE

The Great Pretender

"Look a Little Closer"
Song and lyrics by Nick Ivanovich

I've walked through the forest scarred by fire.
I found myself sinking into a spiritual quagmire.
Oh, I hit bottom like a lead balloon.
I was abandoned and left for dead I assumed.

But look a little closer.
See the start of a new life.
Look a little closer
At what love has revived.
Look a little closer
See a beautiful day.
Look a little closer,
I believe it's gonna be OK.

I was swallowed up, just Jonah.
Tossed around in the belly of life's crazy
    moments.
Walking this scorched and barren land.
I was hungry and thirsty and a broken man.

Jonah and the whale.

"Get out of here!" Mom shrieked every day at the doctors trying to care for her in the psychiatric ward of the Methodist Hospital. They relayed this information to Dad when he called about her.

"She thinks demons are in her room," Doctor Haycraft told Dad. "So just be aware of this when you come to visit."

She had only been in the hospital a few days when we all drove over to see her. She was very different from when we had found her in the park.

"Get out! All of you, get out!" Mom screamed. "The devil is in here, and he wants all of you. You need to leave now!"

She was hysterical with fear. If they had given her any medications to calm her down, it wasn't obvious.

"Linda, honey, it's good to see you," Dad said. He tried to be soft and gentle, as if he were trying to calm a young child.

"No! No! No! It's not safe for any of you!" Mom shouted. "Don't you understand that there's an evil conspiracy going on with the Illuminati? They've signed a pact with the devil, and they have to re-cruit as many souls as possible. You're not safe here!"

Her eyes were wild like those of a wounded animal.

She was Jonah and had been swallowed by the whale.

I started shaking. Grammy grabbed my hand.

"I've had enough of this shit," Rachel said. She turned and walked out the door, back to the lobby.

I looked toward the nurses' station, where two nurses watched us intently. Visitors weren't usually allowed in patients' rooms, but be-cause Mom had been there only a few days, they let us visit briefly.

"Honey, no one is going to take us," Dad said. "We're just here to see you. The girls made you a card." He held out the card that I had painted for Mom. She slapped it out of his hand.

"It's tainted now, don't you see?" she yelled at him. "The devil can get to us through anything."

Dad continued to act like everything was normal. "How are things going? Are you doing OK in here?"

"Get away from me *now*!" she screamed again. Her eyes bulged from her face. She looked like she was seeing the devil himself. "Don't you dare come near me!"

"C'mon, Karena," said Grammy. "Let's go. We're not doing her any good by being here."

"Yes, *go*, Momma, *go!*" Mom screamed at her mother. "Get Karena out of here too!"

A nurse hurried in and recommended that we leave. She observed how Mom was becoming more agitated with us being there.

I couldn't stop shaking.

I needed something to take away this pain and confusion.

I just had to get out of there.

We left the hospital, and I decided to not go back until Mom had stabilized. I couldn't take it anymore.

The doctors put Mom on antipsychotic medication, and in a couple of weeks, her delusions began to melt away. She was stable and coherent. The doctors began preparing Mom to go home.

I was nervous. Rachel was skeptical. Dad was hopeful yet wary too. Grammy just wrung her hands when we talked to her about it. She had lived with my grandfather—Mom's dad—and was well aware of all the traps in believing things would be OK when they really weren't. She was not as hopeful as I was.

I wanted this to work. I wanted Mom to be with us, even if she was broken. I was convinced that love could heal anything, and I loved her with all my heart, although I was often furious with her for abandoning us.

When Dad brought her home, she was *mostly* herself. Her medication was stabilizing, and she was seeing a psychiatrist regularly. But she didn't like the way the medications made her feel and complained constantly. Most of the time, she walked around in her pajamas like a zombie. Her fire was gone. Her spirit and creativity gone. She was a shell of the Mom I knew when I was little. She wasn't delusional, but she was no longer there.

"Nick, I don't like it," Mom said one evening. "I feel like I'm walking through sludge. I can't think. I can't concentrate."

"Maybe we just need to make some adjustments with the medication," Dad said. "You need these meds, Linda. Without them, you're not well. And you can't just stop your treatment plan with your psychiatrist. You need her."

"She doesn't do any good," Mom said. "It's a waste of time."

For a while, Mom took her medication, but then she stopped. She was quiet about her paranoia and suspicions. She could convey a sense of normalcy. She could pretend she was still on medication when she wasn't. But all along, she was becoming more cunning, deceptive, and manipulative. We tried not to notice.

The truth is, sometimes people don't change. Perhaps they *can't* change. Sometimes they get swallowed up by the whale and never get out. They refuse their medications. They refuse psychiatric help. They refuse the love that family members and friends offer. Maybe we can't expect them to change. They just pretend to be a certain way for a while because they're determined to get their way.

We should have seen it coming.

CHAPTER TWENTY-FOUR

The Rave and Handcuffs

Every day is confusing
While I try moving
Past the things that have passed
Abandoned and coming in last
Life trips me up
And every sip from the cup
Of the pleasures I find
Gives me no peace of mind
Not music and drugs, not boys and sex
Forget about Love
Through all this deception
I can't find redemption
My demons are haunting
And I find myself wanting
Of everything.

—Karena, age fourteen

Escapism . . .
    I giggled. Natalie giggled. High already from doing meth and E at
her house, we sped to an abandoned warehouse near Center Run Drive

in downtown Indianapolis in Natalie's father's old, beat-up Toyota truck. It was going to be a typical rave on a Friday night. As long as the party didn't get busted, we would be happy! Tonight's party featured Dru Duncan, a DJ from Chicago. He was one of our favorites. He knew how to help us escape and had earned his reputation in gabber, hardcore, and speedcore. He would serve up a smooth blend of breakbeat and techno, sprinkled with a selection of well-known underground anthems.

In the truck, I experienced waves of dizziness as if I were going to faint. My body was numb but stimulated. My bones ached beyond belief. I just wanted to dance and shake off the ache.

Before we left Natalie's, I'd looked in the mirror and tried to comb my hair. It was long and hanging over my shoulders, and I couldn't get the tangles out. It felt as though my eyes were bulging out of my head. I laughed. My face was hard to recognize. It was pale. Even though I knew it was the effects of the drugs and sadness, at the moment, I didn't care.

At the old warehouse, Natalie parked the truck and we got out. It had rained earlier, and the sidewalks were still wet. The smell of sodden leaves filled the air.

As we walked to the entrance, we wove through a zombie tribe of crackheads spilling from an alleyway, their eyes widened unnaturally from sockets hollowed into sunken faces as if searching for the sleep they probably had not had in days. We tried to avoid contact with them. Even high on meth, I sensed they could be dangerous.

Familiar faces greeted us at the door, which was on the back side of the building, out of view for anyone driving downtown. Natalie and I hugged the regulars. Wes, Chris, Candace, Jonathan, Vickie. Drag queens, club kids, ravers.

Red lights steered us down a corridor and past a room with an overflowing toilet reeking of sewage. Natalie and I ignored it and giggled again. My heart was racing. The whole building was pulsating with energy.

A purple strobe light beckoned, and we vanished into the smoke-machine haze that smelled of burnt cotton candy and lined the insides of our noses with soot.

Guys wore jeans and hoodies; girls had on neon colors, cropped tops, and tie-dyes. It was not just the music we ravers cared about. It was also the fashion. We were rebels. With our motto of *freedom, peace, and love*, we were similar to the hippies of the '60s. We wanted to let go and be free. We were too young for the regular clubs, and we wanted to stand out in our private clubs, which emulated the neon and strobe lighting of club scenes. At a rave, we were free to be whomever we wanted.

Natalie and I moved into the crowds and moshed together, dancing and laughing. Cute boys danced close, and, several times, I kissed the boy in front of me. I didn't know him. I only knew that, at the time, I thought he was very sexy.

We danced for hours to electronic dance music, hypnotic music—trance, tribal, house—mostly without lyrics, except for phrases repeated by strange and otherworldly voices. Voices that often followed me home long after the rave had ended.

The music was amplified by a large, powerful sound system. Sometimes there were laser light shows, projected images on the walls, and fog machines.

Drugs were passed around freely as people zoned out on Ecstasy, meth, cocaine, weed, and ketamine. And more. Plenty more. It was exciting, euphoric, and empowering. Of course, that high never lasted.

Later, I would battle through the crash. During the high, you soared on dopamine levels three times the norm, making you feel superhuman, unstoppable, but when those surplus neurotransmitters were exhausted, your dopamine plummeted and you crashed to earth, drained and depressed.

That night, I stayed over at Natalie's. I'd left a note for Dad so he wouldn't be worried. Many times, I swore never to do meth again, but I went back to it, just like I did with other drugs. Whatever I could find. I could always rationalize fleeing for a few days into the beauty and abandonment of a drug-induced nirvana.

I'd first started going to raves with my friend Graham, a DJ from London. He introduced me to the world of house and techno music—and led me further into the expansive world of drugs. He was dealing on the side, and he also taught me how to sell drugs. It was a great way to earn extra money as well as get my own drugs. I was fourteen when I first kissed Graham. He was eighteen years old, with curly black hair and a beautiful British accent. We were at the apartment of a friend of Graham's, Jonathan. Jonathan was older, about twenty-four. At one point, Jonathan brought out a large amber jar with a black screw top and a label that read: "Cocaine for Jonathan."

Unscrewing the cap, he took a long-handled cotton swab, swished it around in the jar, then pulled it out, covered in crystals. The crystals had a rainbow quality in the lamplight. He gave it to me, so I put it up my nostril and gently rolled it around. Then I repeated the process with a second swab, and possibly a third.

Almost immediately, the room began to glow and took on a lovely coziness, like being in a hobbit's house. The lights looked softer, and I started feeling really, really good. I mean really, really, really good. I looked over at Graham and kissed him again and again. I thought he looked like a movie star.

—

One night, Natalie and I went to a party at Bradley's. He was one of our raver friends, and his parents were gone for the weekend. We planned to bring as many drugs as we could. "I'm bringing Ecstasy," Natalie bragged. "What about you?"

"Cocaine. I met Jack earlier downtown, and he hooked me up." Jack was a dealer I'd become friends with. I was proud that I had connections in the drug world.

"Hey, you ever had sex with Jack?" Natalie asked. She had the hots for Jack. Big-time. For weeks, all she had been talking about was sex, sex, sex. I didn't care what she talked about as long as it wasn't about my mom.

"Nah, he's more like a brother," I said. "But I do have the hots for Daniel. I hope he's at the party tonight."

"He's so cute," said Natalie. "I could totally see you and him together."

As soon as we entered Bradley's house, friends surrounded us. Everyone was talking about the next rave. A keg had been set up in the kitchen, so we filled our plastic cups up with beer. Music blasted from the stereo, and except for in the kitchen, all the lights in the house were turned off.

Natalie and I sat down on the sofa in the living room. I took a baggie from my pocket and spread the cocaine out, like sugar, on the coffee table. Then we both took a straw and began snorting. It felt fantastic. I licked my fingers and rubbed my gums. I didn't want to waste one tiny speck of it.

For a while, I felt this amazing sensation of invincibility, like nothing was beyond reach. I believed I could do anything and everything in the world that I wanted to. Life always seemed better when I was high.

"Why don't we try smoking it?" said Natalie. "Or shooting it up? They say the euphoria is amazing if you shoot it up a vein."

"Maybe later," I said. "I want to get a beer first." Shooting up was the one thing I wouldn't do, but I didn't want to admit that to Natalie.

In the living room, everyone was dancing and time morphed. I'm not sure how long we were there. At some point, Jack showed up, and he and Natalie disappeared into a bedroom. I looked for Daniel but could not find him. *Bummer.*

Suddenly, we heard sirens outside. *Shit.*

"It's the cops!" someone shouted. A neighbor must have called them. This had happened before. Several times, in fact.

I quickly gulped down the rest of my beer, and we all started dumping the drugs wherever we could. In the toilet. Under the bed. In sock drawers. Anywhere, as long as they weren't on our bodies, so we couldn't be charged with possession. Then everyone ran out the back of the house and into the bushes.

We were loud. Some people giggled while others screamed. I tried to stay quiet. Several officers pointed their flashlights in all directions. Of course, they found us. Moments later, my hands were behind my back and I was handcuffed. "You have the right to remain silent. Anything you say can and will be used against—"

"Yeah, yeah," I said. Then I laughed. "I know the drill!"

I was put in the back of a cop car with a guy from the party. I think his name was Ralph. He was busy singing some song that didn't make any sense. He was barely aware of what was happening.

The seat was hard plastic and cold. Someone had once told me they made the car seats like that so it was easy to clean up a variety of bodily fluids.

My hands were cuffed so tightly that I had to lean forward. My hair had been twisted into a messy bun, but somewhere along the way, it had slipped out and was now hanging in my face.

I was coming down from my high and felt nauseated from the beer and coke. My earlier bravado was melting away.

"This is bullshit!" I screamed to the cops, tears streaming down my face.

Mom was at home! What would she do to me when she heard I was arrested? When I'd been in trouble before, she had been on one of her disappearing acts, and I hadn't had to deal with her.

"Quiet back there," one of the cops up front yelled at me.

I started sobbing, and mascara ran down my cheeks.

The guy riding with me in the back seat seemed oblivious to everything that was happening and just smiled at me. *Idiot!*

The cops brought me and all the other partiers to jail. They took my purse and shoes and gave me a sweatshirt, sweatpants, and some socks.

"I'm not a fucking criminal!" I shouted. "I get a phone call, don't I?" I had called Dad when I got picked up by the police before, and he always came to get me. Even if he was out playing music in a bar somewhere, he dropped everything and came.

Ignoring my request, they made me stand in front of a wall for a mug shot. Did I smile? I do remember that they wouldn't let me comb my hair.

Next, I was fingerprinted. I wondered if that ink could be used in my paintings. Maybe I could use the ink on my fingertips to paint a mural on the cell wall. I laughed.

It felt surreal.

I was given a thick gray wool blanket and led to a small and barren holding cell. When they shut the door and locked it, the clink echoed down the hall. A steel toilet sat in one corner. A roll of toilet paper on the floor. A steel bench along a side wall. It looked sterile and was devoid of life. I paced beneath a ceiling vent that blasted cold, icy air into the room. I thought I would freeze to death.

A police officer came to tell me I was allowed one phone call. He opened the door and took me to a phone on the wall at the end of the hallway. I called Dad. His voice was tired but soothing. "Oh, Karena, again? Didn't you learn from the last time?"

"No sermons, Dad, please. Can you come get me?"

"OK," he said.

I was led back to my holding cell, where I sat with my wool blanket, huddled on the cold metal bench. I couldn't stop crying.

When Dad came, I told him I was sorry and that I would never do that again.

"I know," he said.

I felt bad. "Please don't tell Mom."

"We'll see" was all he said.

Later, when I had to go to juvenile court, Dad came with me. Fortunately, he didn't tell Mom about me being arrested or the court date.

I was charged with public intoxication and resisting arrest and sentenced to community service for six months. I had to volunteer with Big Brothers Big Sisters, and it wasn't so bad. I was luckier than some. Others had to do roadside cleanup as their community service and wear those orange vests. I would have died of embarrassment.

I continued to do drugs and have sex and party and skip school. But, from then on, I made sure it was at a place where the cops would not be called so I would not be hauled off to jail again.

I thought I was being careful until one night, when I was about seventeen, I stood outside a retail shop in downtown Indianapolis. I'd just sold Ecstasy to one of my customers. A middle-aged man wearing khakis and a hoodie approached me. At first, I thought he was going to ask me if I had any weed or Ecstasy for sale. Word had spread that I was the person to see outside certain retail shops if someone was looking to get high. But the man didn't beat around the bush. He was forthright about his intentions.

"I know what you're doing," he said.

"What do you mean?" I tried to play innocent.

Part of me knew instantly he was a cop. *Shit!*

I froze. I knew I was in deep shit if found out and didn't know how my father would respond. *Would I go to jail again?*

I just stared at the policeman. "What do you want?" I asked.

"Look, I know what you're doing," he repeated.

"You do?" My heart was in my throat.

"You have to stop what you're doing, young lady," he said. He flashed his badge.

Holy hell! Fucking shit!

Before I could respond, he glanced around to see if anyone was looking and then whispered, "Look, I'm not going to arrest you. I'm going to let you go this time."

"Thank you," I said. I was shaking.

"Just stop this," he said. "It will lead you down a path of destruction."

With that, he turned and walked down the street.

"Thank you, God!" I whispered in a low voice.

I didn't clean up my act from that encounter, but it showed me that God was looking out for me and had a bigger plan. Somewhere. In time. It was part of my road back to faith.

Years later, after I finally stopped using drugs, I would still imagine getting lost in the temporary happiness, the escape. Even when I began cleaning up my life, there were moments I would fantasize about escaping just once more into that halcyon world.

But as time went on, even that stopped. I remembered that undercover cop who had warned me, then let me go. I have often thought he was an angel in disguise. Thank goodness for that, and thank goodness I found healthier, more productive, and creative ways to channel my darker feelings.

If I hadn't eventually stopped the drugs and channeled my energies into positive things, I probably would have become an addict because I was so fragile. I could have become too dependent on the drugs to bring me happiness, as temporary as each high was. And I could have died.

But I still had a long way to go before that epiphany.

There was still plenty of escaping that I needed to do . . . and plenty of hell to experience.

Later, I would learn more about respecting my parents and loving them. I would fully understand the sacrifices that Dad made for me and our family. As a teenager, you're not fully aware of this. And I would learn that even Mom, who was selfish in her mental illness, loved me as much as she could. As much as she was capable of.

Life is always the best teacher.

CHAPTER TWENTY-FIVE

Jane Doe

There is a silence to my soul. I am wet fall leaves under frost. I am opaque white across the moon. I am chilled blood, coldness bringing the synapses of my brain to a standstill. Part of it is pain, yet it is a feeling I am familiar with and can endure if I continue my escapes. This is my winter. I wait impatiently for spring and the chattering of birds.

—Karena, age sixteen

Delusions.

Mom was home, and Dad continued to pretend everything was OK. Or at least he tried to. Things were clearly not all right.

"Why can't we watch television?" I asked him one night.

"Honey, there's a lot of conspiracies on TV right now, and it's best if we don't watch it," Dad said. "There really could be some evil things happening in our world." He stood in the kitchen, making a sandwich, acting as though this was the most normal thing to say in the world. I looked at him as if he had become delusional himself.

Another night, Mom woke Dad up and shouted at him, "Why are you stabbing me?"

"Honey, I'm not stabbing you," Dad said.

Mom ran out of their bedroom, with a blanket and pillow, and into the bedroom where Rachel and I slept.

I sat up. "Mom?"

"Your dad is trying to kill me," she said.

Yet another night, all the windows in our house had been closed, and Rachel complained that it was stifling hot inside. "Why are all the windows shut?"

"Because your mom said the evil spirits would come in if they were open," Dad said.

Only later would I look back and realize that we were all getting pulled into Mom's world. Little by little. Dad thought it was easier to agree with her than to try and reason with her. But all these episodes, along with the fact that she had begun to spend hours alone in her bedroom, should have signaled to us that Mom was becoming delusional.

Not long after the window incident, Mom disappeared once again. She simply walked out of the house at dawn while the rest of us were asleep.

Once again, we called friends and family members, including Grammy.

"Oh, Nick, I am so sorry," Grammy said. "I haven't heard from Linda. I'll call around and see what I can do."

We were used to this, but, this time, the police couldn't find her. No one had seen a woman walking along the side of the road.

Mom was missing again. It would be another six weeks before we heard anything from her or about her. She had become an expert at disappearing, and now she was determined we would not find her.

Even though we'd been through this before, Dad was worried sick.

One day, I was standing in the hallway and heard him talking to Grammy on the kitchen phone.

"I'm afraid that she's hurt . . . or something. Rose, she had no money . . . nothing. Only the clothes on her back."

I ran to my room and flung myself across my bed and cried and cried. *Was Mom really dead? What happened to her?* I could barely breathe. I was sick to my stomach.

Rachel, Dad, and I tried to go on with our everyday activities as if everything were normal, but we also checked with relatives, neighbors, and friends often. We watched the news, hoping for a sign that a woman was picked up walking the streets.

I often huddled with Bear under the covers and cried. My cat curled up on the bed next to me, trying to comfort me. And I continued to have nightmares. The red vampire eyes were still staring at me throughout the night, and the weird clunk-clunk noises still rang out from the attic. The long tree limbs outside banged across the windowpane as if they were trying to get in.

All the while, we heard nothing about Mom.

Nothing.

Until . . .

Dad received a call and motioned us to the phone. He held the receiver away from his ear so we could listen in as we huddled together in the kitchen.

"Is this Nick?" a voice asked.

"Yes, how can I help you?" Dad said.

"Nick, I'm calling from the psychiatric unit at the Bloomington Meadows Hospital, and we have a homeless lady here who says she is Jane Doe."

"Does this mean you've found my wife?" Dad asked. "Is she all right?"

"Yes, yes, she is OK," the nurse said. "Dr. Perry is a psychiatrist here, and he's been treating her. You filed a missing person's report, right?"

Dad said yes.

"She fits the description in your report."

Dad asked how Mom had been found, and the nurse said the police saw her lying in a ditch, thirty miles south of Indianapolis on State Road 37.

"She was shivering in the cold, without a jacket. The police took her to a hospital where she was treated for hypothermia. She wouldn't give anyone her real name, so the doctors asked for a psychiatric evaluation, and she was transferred to us."

The nurse explained that their Jane Doe was stable but urged Dad to not get his hopes up. It might not be her. "After all, she doesn't admit to being married or having children."

"What are you treating her with?" Dad asked.

"We've started her on Haldol, an antipsychotic medication."

Dad thanked the nurse for calling and said he'd be right there. He hung up the phone and told me and Rachel to get in the car. We were going to Bloomington.

I tried to be optimistic along the way but felt tired of the familiar struggle. For years, we'd been teetering between Mom being home with us and Mom abandoning us and becoming a homeless person, a Jane Doe. I was so tired of getting my hopes up that she would get well and become a real mother again. I was so tired of the fear that nothing would ever be right again.

What's wrong with our family? I thought over and over again. I couldn't help but recall our family background and history. For the first time, I was acknowledging that I would have to deal with the mental illness in our family. I longed to bury my head in Mom's chest and feel her arms around me as she stroked my hair and comforted me. *Aren't mothers supposed to do that? Aren't they supposed to be at home with their children, caring for them?* I had not experienced much physical contact from Mom since I was very young. And I was starved for that kind of nurturing.

Mom was so different from what I thought a normal mother should be. Even so, I often wondered if schizophrenia was a "normal" part of life.

WHAT IS REALITY?

*Essay for English Class
by Karena*

What is "real" is merely someone's opinion, taken on naively by all of us. As Americans, we are brought into the world with blinders on. We are raised to live in self-doubt and fear if we do not succeed personally and professionally in a way that society expects, or the way others expect and believe is real.

As a child growing up in the Midwest, I was born with a blueprint of who I was going to be. I was going to be raised a certain way, believe in a certain God, convey a certain personality. I would attend a certain college and pursue a certain major. After college, I would get married, have children, and raise them to be just like me with the same sense of reality.

This reality seems genuine enough, so because it's so genuine, we are tempted to make it an actuality. The reality blueprint becomes our personal reality. This is where we have been deceived. If we do not follow this "blueprint," we are considered "disturbed" and can even be diagnosed with some sort of physical or mental disorder.

Who decided that a person with schizophrenia has a false perception of reality? Their thoughts and lifestyle may be different from what society wants to accept as normal, so we call them crazy. But crazy? Compared to whom?

Any aspect of reality can be examined, scrutinized, and even altered. We are afraid to give ourselves the opportunity to experience something new because it may be judged or seem "off" to someone. We've become unable to admit our true thoughts and feelings to ourselves; therefore, we continue down our same old paths.

As I've searched deeper and deeper within myself to define reality, I've realized that all things that exist are real. Each individual's belief system becomes their personal reality. And whether it's right or wrong, evil or kind, neurotic or otherwise, it is their reality.

As we progress in life, we need to realize that we may never grasp the concept of reality because it's different for everyone. Perhaps it doesn't exist. Perhaps, as humans, we're just looking for some sort of foundation on which we can build our lives. Perhaps we all live in our own world of reality, with our own beliefs of what is, or should be, real.

Just as it should be.

—

Because I had so little affection and love in my life, drugs and sex were part of my escape therapy. Yet I needed to know deeply and intimately what was wrong with everything in my life. My heart had been broken over and over again by Mom. It would only be later that I truly understood how our broken hearts have the potential to open us to a wider sense of identity, and with this realization would come the ability to see through the partitions that separated us from the world. To learn this lesson, I had to rediscover my sense of origin and embrace it. But at that time, I didn't have a clue.

I thought about Babushka and Geed, Dad's mother and father from Ukraine, who were almost murdered by Nazis. I thought about my mom's mother, Grammy. My grandparents loved me and Rachel. *So, what happened to Mom? Didn't she inherit the love gene?* It was clear she didn't love me or any of us. Or perhaps she simply didn't know how to love anymore.

Somewhere along the way, I slowly began to embrace my sense of origin. I began to accept that a mental health disorder is serious and it wasn't Mom's fault. It was in her DNA. Coded in her genes. And it had been there since the origin of her family's DNA. And even though it was difficult for me to accept, I later learned that I would excel because of the lessons involved.

To distract myself from the pain of thinking about Mom, I looked out the window at the scenery of wet roads and hillsides on our way to Bloomington. I also planned how Natalie and I would get to the next rave. The drugs and music were enticing, and I could dance out all my nervous energy.

When we arrived at the hospital, Dad parked the car and we got out. Pulling my jacket tighter around me, I felt the harsh wind rustle through my hair. I didn't want to cry, worried that the tears would freeze on my cheeks.

None of us said anything as we went through the entry. The sterile white hallways were daunting. Scary and empty. The sounds of doors slamming shut and clinking metal locks rang out in the distance, reminding me of horror movies with psych wards as in *One Flew Over the Cuckoo's Nest*. Nurse Ratched might come around the corner at any moment, a hatchet in her hand, staring at us with cold, heartless eyes.

My whole body shook with dread.

After Dad explained who we were at reception, the nurse told us that Jane Doe was in room 103. Like programmed robots, we marched silently to her room.

Dr. Perry met us there and described the situation further. "At first, we couldn't get any information out of her, but once she started taking Haldol, she admitted that she has a husband and children."

"Did she say anything else?" Dad asked.

"She said she'd disappeared once before but got back in touch with you and moved back home. Other than that, she won't tell us much."

I did not want to go into that room. But I needed to see for myself. I looked at Rachel, and she nodded. I knew she felt the same way. We both needed to know.

Dr. Perry unlocked the door. I heard that metal clinking sound again.

My heart was in my throat.

Part of me was screaming for us to turn around.

Dad waited for me and Rachel to step inside first. A woman sat upright on a twin bed in the far corner of the room. She stared straight ahead and didn't even turn our way. Her long dark hair was familiar, but now it looked like the stringy hair of a witch. Even from the doorway, I could tell that the hospital gown she had on was faded and worn. She tugged at the blanket around her shoulders. A small lamp sat on the table beside her bed, casting a dark-yellow glow over the room.

Jane Doe turned and looked at us, her face appearing ghostly with shadows in the light. My heart sank.

"Hi, Nick." Her voice was blank. Hollow.

Dad turned to Dr. Perry. "That's my wife, Linda."

She said hello to me and Rachel, but there was no sign of warmth. Her eyes were vacant, her body rigid.

—

Mom was once again diagnosed with paranoid schizophrenia. Same diagnosis as before, but for whatever reason, it seemed more official this time. More serious. More final.

"I've told your wife this," said Dr. Perry, "but it's important that you know too. Her psychosis from the schizophrenia will probably come back to haunt her countless times for the rest of her life. The medication I'm giving her should stabilize her, but it might take some time, and we have no way of knowing whether she will have more psychotic episodes."

"I understand," said Dad. "We just want to take her home, Doc."

Mom looked disinterested as Dr. Perry talked. He explained how there was a mandated legal hold on Mom. Once she was stabilized, the hospital could ask the court to turn her over to Dad legally so he could get psychiatric care for her.

Not long after that, the police escorted Mom to the courthouse for a hearing. The judge determined that Dad could bring her home, but she had to continue her medications and undergo psychiatric treatment with monthly visits to her psychiatrist.

I knew that I would have to find a way to be understanding and loving toward a mother who had hurt me time and time again. It seemed like a lot for a teenager to manage. But I would try. And I had the drugs, the parties, and my art, which helped me escape.

At night, my reality warped into nightmares and red vampire eyes. I couldn't escape my dreams where the demons haunted me.

CHAPTER TWENTY-SIX

Homecoming

The emptiness is always there; I consider myself
    an expert
at hiding it. Wildness runs through my veins.
No one will know while I'm smiling. It hides
    everywhere, this
emptiness . . . in the closet, the cabinets . . . in my
    art.
There isn't any getting away from it, though. The
    emptiness is like those vampire
eyes that are always in my window at night. I'm so
    fucking scared of them, but
I cannot get rid of them. And I need to feel some-
    thing. Anything.
I need those vampire eyes to distract myself from
    being so lonely and empty.

—Karena Dawn

Spotless.

I wanted the house to be spotless. The doctor told Dad that the Haldol had stabilized Mom and she had been doing well in her psychiatric sessions. Mom was coming home!

Rachel thought I was being dumb, but she didn't understand. I wanted Mom to feel happy that she was home. A clean house would be inviting and make her feel good. I scrubbed the bathrooms and floors with bleach until my fingers were raw. I dusted every picture and knickknack on our bookshelves. I washed the bedsheets so her bed would smell fresh, and I set up an easel with paints in the basement. Mom was a brilliant artist, and I hoped that if she could get back to it, it would help with her problems.

"Look, Karena," said Rachel, "Mom isn't *fixed*. The meds only stabilize her, but she's still the same selfish person she has always been. Don't get your hopes up."

"I know," I said, throwing Rachel a mean look. "But I'm going to give her a chance. She deserves that."

Rachel shrugged. "I really don't care."

When Dad pulled up in the driveway, I ran out to greet them. Mom got out of the car, wearing the jeans and sweater Dad had taken to the hospital. She smiled.

"Hello, Karena."

"Mom, I'm so glad you're home!" I ran to her and put my arms around her. She returned the hug, and I ignored how she was stiff and standoffish. We went inside.

"Karena cleaned the house for you," Dad said. "Doesn't it look nice?"

"Mmm . . . oh, sure," Mom said. "It looks nice, Karena." She managed a small smile, and that little smile made me hopeful. Mom had come and gone through the years, but maybe, this time, with the right medication and therapy, her moods would stabilize and she'd be part of our family again.

"Hi, Rachel," Mom said.

"Umm, hi." Rachel was cold. Detached.

The first few weeks were almost normal. I stayed at the house more after school instead of partying so much on weekdays. Dad scheduled an appointment for me and Rachel to see a therapist, and we went to one session, but neither of us would talk. Life was too *private* for me to share with a therapist at that time.

Things became routine.

Wake up. Shower. Throw on my school clothes.

Go downstairs and notice that Rachel has already left for the day.

Eat breakfast with Mom in the kitchen while we sit silently.

Try to ignore Mom, telling myself she is "mostly" normal.

Love the feeling of being high.

Life is blissful . . . for a while.

Go to art class. Teacher encourages me to become a great artist.

Love my art class.

Skip lunch.

Come home.

Make small talk with Mom. Watch her carefully to see if she's acting normal.

Dinner with Dad and Mom, and sometimes Rachel.

Go to bed.

Hear tree limbs scratching on the window. And noises in the attic, sometimes, not always.

Hear Mom and Dad arguing.

Begin to hear Mom screaming.

Hell no.

Have nightmares all night long.

On weekends, I stayed out very late, going to parties, doing drugs, and hanging out with my friends. I sometimes visited New Age People to meditate, hoping to see the White Tiger again or meet the wolf inside.

Mom didn't seem to notice when I was gone. Neither did Dad. Or, if they noticed, they didn't care.

As before, I desperately wanted the mom back that I had known as a little girl, but it was becoming obvious that she was gone and never returning. And, as usual, Dad tried to act as though everything was OK.

But it wasn't long before I saw the cracks in Mom's behavior, and in her thinking, again. She wanted to save us. And, this time, she told me I could go with her when she left. "That way, I know you'll be safe from the apocalypse that's coming. And safe from the demons of your father."

"But, Mom," I said, "why do you want to leave? You have everything you need right here. You have us. And Grammy. We're your family."

Mom would look at me like I was naive and uninformed about the true ways of the world.

She remained somewhat stable for a while, continued taking her medication, and even returned to work as a social worker in an assisted-living facility, helping individuals who suffered from age-related mental illness.

"Rose, it's ironic, if you ask me. Here she is, barely functioning, and she's now got a job helping others!" Dad was on the phone with Grammy.

Grammy thought maybe it would be good for her to help others instead of focusing on herself so much. That made sense to me.

Mom would often say, "I don't have any schizophrenic thoughts today and I don't feel like I'm on any medication."

I loved it when Mom said those things.

But after a few months, she began to struggle with accepting her disorder. And then, at one of her visits to her psychiatrist, Mom asked him to take her off the medications on a trial period because she was doing so well. Much to Dad's chagrin, the psychiatrist did just that.

"The legal hold has expired," Dr. Haber said when Dad complained. "Before, it was a mandated treatment by the courts that Linda be on medication, but that hold has expired, and there's nothing I can do if she wants to go off it."

"I don't think she's strong enough," Dad said. "She's been through this before. She gets better and seems normal and goes off the meds, and then it's not long before she disappears."

"Sorry, Nick, but that's the law."

—

Dad later told me that once Mom was off the medication, he started noticing her transition into delusional thoughts again. "It was almost like I accepted her delusions as normal at first," he told me. "I accepted her warped thinking."

We stopped watching television again because Mom thought there was too much evil on TV. She was persuasive about her ideas, the way cult leaders could be with their followers. Mom was able to con me and Dad into her way of thinking. She had tried to be a normal mom to me and Rachel and a regular wife to Dad for a while, but the cracks in her behavior grew into chasms day by day. Mom was suspicious of everything. She worried about the food we ate, the clothes we wore, the books we read. The psychosis sometimes seemed like a bad fever that came and went. Sometimes she fixated on religion; other times, she was intensely paranoid and delusional. Whenever Mom was off her meds, she was a stranger in our house and we were all helpless to her illness.

When, as an adult, I asked Dad about his marriage to Mom, he told me that their marriage was nothing like he had expected. He kept thinking she would get better, just like I did. And when Mom didn't get better, he tried to normalize her behavior. He even tried to accept it when she would wake up in the middle of the night, screaming at him. Or when she demanded that the windows stay closed so evil spirits couldn't come in. Dad knew it wasn't normal, but he tried to make life feel normal and routine for me and Rachel.

Dad's music sustained him. But I know he was frustrated and lonely. Just like I was. And Rachel too. Our lives were stripped down to the barest essence of survival. I had my drugs and wild parties. I had my art. Rachel had her own world of friends, and she had her poetry. We were all artists, and creativity helped us.

We didn't know who Mom was going to be from day to day. It was always a guess when she woke up each day and when Rachel and I came home from school. Would she be normal? Or would she be paranoid and delusional, believing demons were coming to get us? What would her reality be that day?

We never knew. We all tried to be hopeful, but it was difficult.

But no matter what, I knew I could not give up hope. If I did, I would die.

CHAPTER TWENTY-SEVEN

Kiss Me Goodbye

"The Road"
Poem by Rachel Sahaidachny

and the woman and the road
and the road and the woman in her car
with her dog and the road
and her dog and her breath
and the lots and parks in dark
sleeping in her car
and the woman and her dog
living in her car
and the woman who believes
who flees past town and suburbia
and the woman flees tourist nation
and believes everything is fake
and believes she is OK living
in her car with her dog

all night I dreamed about shit and piss
I dreamed about leaking from my guts
I woke up burning in my head
it's always the same
as though inside I hold a locket of memories

staring across the vast country
threading my brain to her flash
all night on the road
the woman and her dog
gray mirrors on pavement and sky
of her eyes always peering into her lord
peering into suffering attached
vast expanses peering at her
gray pavement peering at stoplights
suffering signals that say Don't Walk
holding on to steering wheel
her eyes mirrored in the rearview
it's always the same

Kisses.

In November 1998, Mom had worked the entire weekend. She had Monday off, but she got up and made coffee and a piece of toast for breakfast. Rachel and I went to school. Everything seemed as normal as it could be.

As Dad got ready for work, Mom sat in a chair in the den, staring out the window with her coffee in hand. He told her he'd see her that evening and to enjoy her day off. When Mom asked if he was going to kiss her goodbye, it seemed a little odd. She was seldom affectionate. Most of the time, she didn't even sleep in their bedroom; rather, she slept on the floor in my and Rachel's room or on the sofa downstairs. He gave her a kiss; maybe it was going to be a good day after all. After the kiss, Mom just looked at him with a half smile and said nothing.

—

Mom had always been rigid and harsh, even when we were younger. When she'd become vegetarian, so did the rest of the family. When she started eating meat again, she expected us to do the same and would punish us harshly for not eating the turkey and chicken she cooked. "This is how I show my love," she said.

I kept a little bag packed in my closet so I could run away if I had to.

Mom often yelled at us for no reason. There was the time I helped Rachel get ready for the prom. I wasn't old enough to go to prom, but Rachel was, and I was excited for her. I braided her hair and twisted it on top of her head. We both beamed when we looked at it in the mirror.

When Rachel's date arrived, Mom screamed that Rachel could not leave the house with her hair that way. When Rachel shouted back, Mom grabbed her by the arm and dragged her to the bathroom. "You have to take that hair down *now*!"

I started crying. "Mom, I think it looks great on Rachel!"

Rachel yelled, "Leave me alone! I can wear my hair the way I want to!"

"Take your hair down now or I will take it down for you!" Mom screamed again.

Rachel's date stood at the front door, helpless.

I felt so bad for Rachel. With her mascara streaming down her cheeks, her hair now falling around her shoulders, she ran to the front door, grabbed her date, and left the house.

I went to my room and cried more.

Two years later, during my junior year in high school, Mom and I went shopping for a prom dress for me. I didn't have a date. I was going with a group of friends. But, while shopping, Mom told me that I couldn't buy anything trashy. I shot back, "Look, it's my prom, and I'll buy whatever I want!"

I was grounded for talking back and couldn't go to the prom. I hated Mom for that. Rachel had warned me that I "talked back" too much and it would get me in trouble.

So Mom acting rigid didn't set off any alarm bells.

—

I came home from school that day, wondering what we were going to have for dinner. To my surprise, Mom was standing at the door, waiting for me. A suitcase was behind her on the floor.

"Karena, I'm going to leave, and I want to take you with me."

"What?"

"I can't stay here any longer, but I want you to come with me. You're not safe here. I've been trying to warn you."

I started crying.

"You can pack a few things to bring with you, but don't pack anything with images on it. That's how the demons attach themselves to you."

I just looked at her.

"Oh, and I'll get us some food to take with us." She turned and headed toward the kitchen.

Doesn't she see that I'm crying? Doesn't she realize I have school?

I immediately called Dad. "Mom's planning to leave, and she wants to take me with her!"

"What the hell?" Dad screamed. He sounded hysterical. "Where's she going?"

"I don't know, Dad. But she told me to pack my things."

"Karena, you stay put. Do not go anywhere. And try to keep her there too. I'm coming home," Dad said.

I knew he was about twenty-five miles from our house, so it would take him at least a half hour to get there. Somehow, I had to stall Mom and keep her from going. I started to look for the keys to our extra car.

"Karena, you ready?" Mom came out of the kitchen with a small paper bag and the keys in her hand. I knew I wouldn't be able to get those keys from her.

"Mom, I can't go," I said, wiping my eyes. "I've got school, and I—I—I just can't go."

"Look, you're not safe here, Karena," she said. "Nick is going to brainwash you. He's in on the conspiracy."

I shook my head. "No, Mom, he isn't!"

"Fine!" Mom shouted. She grabbed her suitcase, went out the door, and slammed it behind her.

"Mom, where are you going?" I yelled after her.

But she was already in the car and pulling out of the driveway.

I tried to call Rachel but couldn't get in touch with her.

When Dad got home, I was curled up in a fetal position on the sofa, sobbing. Mom had just ripped my heart out once again.

He ran over and hugged me. "It's all right, Karena," he said. "We'll find her. We always do. And she might even come home tonight or in a couple of days. We've been through this before."

I nodded, but this time, I had a feeling her leaving might be for good.

Dad called Grammy.

He discovered that Mom had not only taken the spare car but also emptied the family's bank account. He called the police and gave them a description of the automobile. We checked all the hospitals and emergency rooms. She became a missing person once again.

Nothing came up in the search until Dad received a phone call from a police officer in Effingham, Illinois, about a week later. Just west of Indianapolis, the police officer had found Mom's wallet and ID. At that point, the police issued an all-points bulletin for her in that area and said they'd call Dad back in twenty-four hours. When they did, they said they couldn't locate her.

Months went by, and none of us heard anything from her. Dad called the National Alliance on Mental Illness and enlisted their help in looking nationwide for Mom. The gentleman at NAMI told Dad, "We're sorry to hear what you're going through. We're going to put some volunteers together to help look for your wife." Dad had sent them a photo of Mom, and it was distributed in police cars across the country.

We heard nothing for an entire year.

Then, one day, Dad got a phone call out of the blue from a former coworker of Mom's. She said she thought she knew where Mom might be. Mom had just used the woman's name as a work reference and had given the address of a women's shelter in Santa Monica, California, as her place of residence.

She gave Dad the name of the shelter. He called and spoke to the psychiatrist there, contacted an attorney in LA, and flew out to California to talk to Mom.

Dad met his attorney at the shelter, and together they talked to the police, the coordinator at the shelter, and the psychiatric team. The attorney had already prepared the papers for Dad, but the shelter coordinator said the papers needed to be drawn up in Los Angeles County.

Dad tried to explain. "She's my wife, she's a mother, and she was employed back home in Indiana," he told them. "And then she just got up one day and walked out. She also left her psychiatric care at home. I have all the paperwork to substantiate that."

The coordinator said that Mom had the right to refuse treatment and to refuse to see Dad. She also said Mom was "a model resident" who'd told them she did not want to go home.

Dad was crushed, but there was nothing he could do about it, according to the police.

Tears welled up in Dad's eyes as he recounted the story to me once he was back home. "I was so frustrated and discouraged. The police in LA were sympathetic and told me they knew I was hurting. They seemed very sincere. They even talked to Linda and tried to persuade her to see me, but she said no."

He looked into the distance as he continued. "Karena, I stood on the street corner in Santa Monica, and I saw all these homeless people begging for food. I just hope that Linda doesn't end up out there on the streets like those other people."

That night, I sobbed. *Mom doesn't love me enough to come home!* She had always come home before. But not this time. And now she was two thousand miles away.

By then, Rachel was already in college at Indiana University and didn't care whether Mom was home. When I talked to her about how hard Dad had tried, she just said, "I can't believe he put up with her for this long."

As for Dad, he was finally over it. He had suffered long enough. He began divorce proceedings. He had done everything in his power to get Mom back, but she had refused. He wanted Rachel and me to know he'd tried his very best.

Our home became a cold, lonely place. Dad worked through the day and most evenings, and the house felt hollow. Lifeless. Our beautiful two-story Tudor house seemed like a morgue.

I could not bear the sadness and loneliness that hung in the air. The memories—both good and bad—echoed off every wall, in every corner. So I also stayed away as much as possible. Now and then, Rachel would invite me to Indiana University for the weekend, and I enjoyed that. But I mostly continued to be rebellious, diving deeper into the rave scene, dancing my pain away. When I wasn't out partying, I was alone. I didn't even see Grammy anymore, now that Mom was gone.

As always, I turned to my journal.

> *Mom is gone. Really gone. It's over. In my sadness there is no past or future, just heavy footsteps, living moment to moment. Every day is measured from the moment of waking into this new reality until my body can do no more, until sleep comes, and even then, the nightmares prevail. Each day I greet the sun like a mountain climber greets their rope, fingers holding on fast until chafed and sore, despite the pain.*
>
> *This is my grief, coming in wintry waves. It is abandonment that flows through my veins and deadens my heart. It is a poison to my spirit, dulling all other emotions. It is as if a black mist had settled upon me, and no matter how bright the day is, I feel no sun and hear no bird song. Only the drugs, partying, sex, and rebellion can bring the real me back into focus. Without them, I will die.*

Dad and I were two lonely souls. Drifters who had very little to anchor us in this world. We both dealt with the pain in our separate ways. Dad had his music. I had my wildness.

I finally graduated from high school and enrolled in Indiana University.

But I never made it to IU.

California was beckoning . . .

PART SIX

California

CHAPTER TWENTY-EIGHT

The City of Angels

"Look a Little Closer"
Song and lyrics by Nick Ivanovich

Look a little closer,
See the start of a new life.
Look a little closer
At what love has revived.
Look a little closer,
See the start of a beautiful day,
Look a little closer,
I believe it's gonna be OK.

Look a little closer, look a little closer,
See the beginning of a new life,
Look a little closer,
At the moon shining bright,
Look a little closer,
I believe it's gonna be all right.

God.

The sunset was dazzling in its brilliance, a million diamonds flung across the ocean waves with gossamer-thin angel wings lightly covering blue. I held my breath, floating numb in captivity of this grandeur. It was so beautiful, I ached. This was my God.

This is how I felt when I watched my first sunset on the beach in Santa Monica. I was in heaven. A world away from gray, wintry, lonely Indianapolis. Already, it felt as though the weight of the last several years of pain and heartache had lifted.

The ocean was just as I had envisioned it—vast and powerful, each wave crowned with sea foam. I threw off my shoes and let my feet sink into the soft, warm sand. I waved at my friend Julie, who was standing behind me. We had arrived at LAX, rented a car, and driven straight to the beach.

"C'mon, Julie! The sand is wonderful!" I felt happy in another world. *California. I'm a Cali girl!*

Julie kicked off her shoes and ran toward me.

"Ooh, it's so soft," she said.

Both of us in jean shorts, we sat down on the beach, feeling the warm sun on our legs and faces. People were laughing and running across the sand. Nearby, a group played volleyball. All were oblivious to the reality of snow and cold back in the Midwest.

The ocean breeze whispered into my ears, sweet like a lover, placing salty kisses on my cheek and tousling my long brown hair. I stretched out my arms and hands, letting the warmth of the sun wrap around my fingers. The warmth of that lazy, carefree breeze was just a mere hint of its power. I believed it had the strength to restore happiness to my heart and soul. I had been so cold for so long.

I wasn't sure how Julie was doing, but when I glanced over at her as she lay on the beach, her smile told me that she felt the same. California was a beautiful world. And the warm breeze whispered of only sweetness and joy.

I couldn't wait until I learned how to surf and became a part of this California lifestyle.

—

By the time Julie and I arrived for our visit in California, Mom had left the shelter where she was staying, gotten another job in social work, and moved into a small one-bedroom apartment in Hollywood. This was typical of her. When she was stable, she could always find a job. And when she did, she reminded me of the Mom I had when I was a child.

By now, Mom and Dad were officially divorced, but that hadn't stopped me from hoping she would come back home to Indianapolis. After Dad told me they had divorced, I was a mess. I felt fully abandoned. Discarded. I'd felt for years that Mom didn't love me or want to be around me, but the divorce made it feel so much more final.

I was restless. Despair filled me at every turn, heavy and suffocating. For a while, I stumbled around in Indianapolis, going to even more raves, and pressing forward until my soul was worn to the bone.

Mom had called me at home from time to time, and when I told her I missed her, she urged me to come out to California after graduation before starting college at Indiana University. I began to think that maybe going to California would help lift my depression. Mom told me that I would love the beach and sunshine. The more I thought about it, the better it sounded.

Because I hated high school so much, I took night classes and graduated early, in January of my senior year. I told Dad I was going to California to visit Mom. I'd be starting college in the fall. He didn't think it was a good idea, but once I told him that my friend Julie would go with me, he relented. Julie and I had met while working at a retail store in Indy and had become fast friends after I'd learned that she enjoyed drugs and raves as much as I did. We both had heard about the amazing raves in California.

When I turned seventeen, Dad had cosigned for a sporty black Acura Integra for me—which I loved with all my heart. I felt so cool in my new car and wanted to drive it to LA, but Dad wouldn't let me. "It's too dangerous and you're too young," he said. "You and Julie can fly."

"But it's expensive to fly, Dad."

"I'll help you with the fare. I'll feel much better about you going to California if you fly."

I was fine with that because we would have more time in California.

In the back of my mind, I naively thought I could convince Mom to come home with me if I went out to visit her. I thought if I talked to her, I could get her to come back to Indianapolis and everything would return to normal. Even though she and Dad were divorced, they would make up and fall in love again. She would once again be a mom to me and Rachel, even though Rachel was already away at college and I would be heading to IU in the fall. Some part of me was still a little girl, wanting Mom to be like all the *good* moms out there in the world. Wanting her to hold me and tell me things would be all right.

Julie and I couldn't wait to see the beach, so after we landed, we rented a car and drove into Santa Monica, maneuvering our way through the traffic. We parked the rental and spent our first couple of hours in California on the beach. After that, we drove to Mom's little apartment in Hollywood.

I was nervous but excited. I had not seen her in a long while.

I knocked on the door. When Mom opened it, my heart lurched. It *was* Mom! I fell into her arms for a hug. She pulled away and smiled.

"Hello, Karena."

"Hi, Mom." Tears filled my eyes, and, at first, I wanted to cry. Then I wanted to scream at her for abandoning us. But I stopped myself and remembered that I was in LA to have a good time and talk her into coming home with me.

When I introduced Mom to Julie, Mom was sheepish about the size of her place and the sparse furnishings.

Julie and I looked around. I had warned Julie beforehand that there probably wouldn't be any furniture—each time Mom ran away from home and got an apartment, she lived without furniture. It reminded me that Mom was never *permanent* anywhere she lived. That it was only a place to stay for a little while. That her illness would tell her to leave, that people were after her, and that she needed to move on. Even though I'd just arrived, it was sinking in that Mom would probably not come back to Indianapolis with me.

"The hotel I booked for you isn't far from here in Santa Monica. It's close to the Third Street Promenade because I assumed you'd enjoy being in that area."

"Thanks, Mom," I said. "Is your job close by?"

"Yes, it's in Santa Monica too, so we can visit after I get off work."
Julie and I thanked Mom for her help.

"I want you girls to have a good time," she said.

Mom told Julie about her job as a social worker. Julie listened politely.
I had only told her a little bit about Mom. Not all the truly awful stuff.

I had to admit, though, it was good to see Mom. The connection
between mother and daughter is stronger than any pain or hurt. And
at the moment, Mom seemed *normal*. Her blue eyes were clear, her
body was healthy looking, and her dark hair was washed and shiny.
Normal. She looked so pretty. I breathed a sigh of relief. Mom was
doing well, I hoped.

A little voice nagged at me, though. I had been through this before,
and I knew Mom was an excellent actress. Nothing was ever truly *normal* with Mom.

While Julie and I stood there making small talk with my schizophrenic mother, my mind wandered to the beach and the beautiful
golden sun. I was so excited about being in California, I decided not to
worry about Mom. Julie and I were there to party and have fun.

After saying bye to Mom and promising that we would visit the
next day when she got off work, Julie and I drove to the small hotel
where we had a reservation. There was nothing fancy about it, but it
was clean with double beds and a shower. That's all we needed.

I called Dad from a pay phone to let him know we had arrived
safely. (It was 1999, so people did not carry cell phones like they do
today.) I told Dad that Mom looked really good, that she had been nice
to me and Julie and seemed stable.

"That's good, Karena," he said. "I hope you girls have a wonderful
time, just be careful. And be cautious around your mom. You know
how she is."

"I know, Dad," I said. "But don't worry. We'll be okay. Mom seems
fine."

"Love you, Karena."

"Love you too, Dad."

Julie and I spent most of our time in Santa Monica by the beach.
It was a place filled with beautiful people. Lean, muscled boys with
sandy blond hair and bikini-clad girls who looked like starlets. Happy

people, smiling. People walking their dogs. People roller-skating and, of course, surfing.

During the day, Julie and I swam in the ocean and dried off on the beach by the pier, or we visited some of the numerous shops and restaurants. We met a couple of cute guys who were street performers on the Promenade. One was Skye, a dancer, and the other was Jeff, who invited us to a rave in Pomona. I was attracted to Skye. He had nice dark eyes, a mop of brown hair, and a strong, athletic body, which he attributed to dancing and surfing. Jeff and Skye were both originally from Michigan, just one state north of ours. Luckily, Julie and Jeff were attracted to each other as well. We were the perfect foursome.

Julie and I were excited about going to the rave that evening. Even though we had been to many raves back home, we'd heard the scene in LA was unlike any other social or music scene in the country. It was grassroots and inclusive and utterly original. And all of this made it intoxicating to be a part of.

As Skye said, "LA is the trailblazer for dance music everywhere in America." And I believed it.

The four of us were inseparable to the point that we didn't really need our hotel room. I stayed with Skye in an apartment in Venice, where he was sleeping on someone's pullout couch, and Julie stayed with Jeff in another friend's apartment.

After being in LA for a week, Julie flew back home as planned. I wanted to stay, so I changed my airline ticket to spend another week with Skye. It seemed as if everyone I met was from somewhere else. People were coming to California to pursue their dreams; it was like no other place in the world, and that was a wonderful thing.

I didn't see much of Mom, but it was OK because she spent most of her time working and seemed quite detached from me. She also appeared to be stable in her life, and I was happy about that.

After two weeks, it was time for me to head back to Indianapolis, back to my retail job and planning for freshman year at Indiana University. But I didn't want to go. I was crazy about Skye and had made new friends. I was already a *California girl*!

Sadly, I knew that I had to go back, though. And I'd accepted that Mom would not come home with me. She was beginning to build a life for herself in California.

When it was time for goodbye, she hugged me and said that if I ever wanted to move to California, I could stay with her.

"Maybe I will," I said. "I really do love it here."

"I think you'd love *living* here too," she said. "You can stay with me, Karena, until you find a job."

Interesting idea, I thought. *Could I live with Mom? Would this give us the opportunity to reestablish our relationship more intimately as mother and daughter? Could I re-create my life in Cali? Maybe the ocean could finally bring me the happiness I was seeking.*

I spent the rest of the day packing my things and imagining what it would be like to live with Mom. Surely it would help mend old wounds, I decided. To have Mom around would be awesome, and I could stay at her place just part-time and spend the rest of my time with Skye. And then, once I found a job and earned some money, I could get my own place but still be near her so we could do daughter-mom things together. Shopping. Getting our hair and nails done. Eating out at restaurants. It could be wonderful.

First, I'd have to talk to Dad about not going to IU *and* moving in with Mom. And I'd have to get things ready for a big move. I couldn't wait. There was something about being in Los Angeles that felt different from anything I had ever experienced before. It was freedom. Creativity. Hope. It was a culture that encouraged creative people to reach for their dreams, whether they were writers, actors, musicians, artists, or builders.

I could barely wait for the time of my departure so that I could return just as fast. And as my plane flew eastward over the golden hills of California, my mind filled with more thoughts about moving and all the possibilities of a new life as I headed into my adult years. And all the possibilities of forging a new relationship with Mom. If I could reclaim her love anywhere, surely it would be in the City of Angels.

CHAPTER TWENTY-NINE

A Little Dream

"Kick the Dust Off Your Shoes"
Song and lyrics by Nick Ivanovich

This road life takes us down
Is marked by blood and tears I have found.
Raise me up from the ashes and rubble.
Shelter me in the day of trouble.

And I bring good news.
Just kick the dust off your shoes
And move on.

Sometimes the darkness grows.
As if God's eyes just closed.
And as I move about this hostile place
I keep my eyes fixed on your face.

And I bring good news.
Just kick the dust off your shoes
And move on.

Sometimes it's hard to relate
At life's every twist of fate.

But when there's a dream like mine
It will all come together in time.

And I bring good news.
Just kick the dust off your shoes
And move on.

Dreamer.

I was ready. To pursue my dreams: to go to California and become
... *what*? I wasn't sure. But I knew one thing: I would turn my dreams
into reality.

When I landed back in Indiana, I was refreshed, excited about life
again, and nearly invincible. I felt giddy with possibilities. Once home,
I couldn't sit down, couldn't read a book, couldn't be still. My mind
was like a butterfly, flitting through the universe. Each time I thought
about LA, I'd get tingly all over.

I wasn't sure how Dad would respond, so I didn't mention my idea
of moving to Los Angeles until after I'd been back home for a couple
of days.

He was scrambling eggs at the stove when I finally brought it up.
He stopped and turned around to look at me, sitting at the kitchen
table, nibbling on a piece of toast.

"What did you say?" He held the spatula in the air like he might
throw it at any moment.

"I want to move to Los Angeles," I repeated, trying to be as non-
chalant as possible. Like it was no big deal.

"Now?" He set the spatula down and removed the skillet from the
burner.

"Yes, now. I can live with Mom."

"Karena, what the hell do you think you're doing? You can't do
that!"

"Why not?" I avoided his eyes. When I did look, I saw pain. It was
clear he didn't want to lose me. Rachel was gone. Mom was gone. I was
the only one left.

"Is this because of your mother? Did she talk you into coming out there and living with her? Karena, you know you cannot trust her. And besides, you're already enrolled in school at IU and you need a college education!" Dad yelled.

"But I don't want to go to IU. I'll go somewhere in LA. I looked into it. I can get my residency after a year, and then school is more afford-able. I don't want to stay here anymore, Dad. It's not you. It's just that LA is so warm and beautiful and fun."

He shook his head, then folded his arms.

"You're only seventeen, Karena. You're still under my roof. You are still a dependent. If you go, I'll take your car away from you. I'll cut you off, and you won't get one more dime from me!"

"I'll be eighteen in March, and besides, I've been making my own car payments," I screamed. "You can't take that car from me."

"Where will you live, Karena?"

"I'm going to move in with Mom."

Dad shook his head. "Your mom's apartment is only two blocks from Hollywood Boulevard, and that's a very dangerous, seedy area."

"I'm going, Dad."

"And, Karena, she'll disappoint you again. She'll break your heart. She has done this over and over again."

"She seems stable, Dad. She goes to work every day." I wanted so much to believe what I was saying was true.

He sighed. "You don't have enough money for a move like this."

"I have my job in the clothing store at the mall, and I'll get a second job as a telemarketer. It pays ten dollars an hour," I said. "I can save up for a couple of months. That money will support me until I find a job in LA."

"Karena, don't you know that LA is a cultural wasteland? It's vapid, flimsy, shallow, and soulless. You'll get swallowed up out there."

"You're wrong," I shot back. "It's beautiful. The people are friendly and creative, and I've never felt so free and happy in my life."

We argued and argued.

But my mind was made up.

I was done with Indiana.

I had new dreams to pursue.

I would listen to the White Tiger.

I would listen to my heart.
I would listen to the calling of a dreamer.
Besides, I had fallen in love with Los Angeles. *The angels.*

CHAPTER THIRTY

Wanderlust

Sissy, you better be good in LA.
I love you and I want to make sure
you write and all. Be good and have a good time.
Watch out for boys and waves and sand.
I'm not gonna lie. I'm gonna worry about you and
wish I could be closer.

Love, Rachel
(letter from college)

Money.

I was proud of myself. I had saved $600 from my telemarketing and retail jobs for my move to Los Angeles. That was big money. Because I had worked so hard at my jobs, Dad finally surrendered and said that he would support my move to LA. He knew I was going either way, so he figured he couldn't clip my wings. I had always been (and still am) a determined person. But there was one condition. Dad and his friend Daniel, who played music with him, were going to follow me out there to make sure I arrived safely.

Rachel seemed genuinely sad and worried that I was moving to California. I laughed and told her that she could come and visit me, and she said she would. She and I had been through so much as children. We shared a unique bond, and no matter if we chose different life paths in different states, we would always have that bond. She was my Sasha and I was her Sissy.

—

Dad later told me that he was sick with worry about me moving to LA. He was concerned that I would never go to college. It was very difficult for him to see me move so far away. He wanted to protect me. He believed I was moving into a very toxic situation with Mom. Of course, I had these worries too, but being only eighteen years old, I was more optimistic. Youth has a way of coloring life in a light that adults can't always see. Although, now that I am older, that optimistic spark is still in me. I was in love with the beach and the sun and believed everything would be OK. But Dad's confidence in the situation was not very high. He also told me years later that there was one thing he'd vowed with all his heart: since he loved me more than life itself, he would do whatever he could to have an ongoing relationship with me and not lose touch. I didn't know this for many years.

—

I had convinced a friend of mine, Kellie, to move to California with me. She was into raves and partying and would be the perfect companion.

We piled our suitcases into my Integra, and Dad and Daniel packed our other belongings into a U-Haul trailer, which they pulled behind Dad's car. With both cars filled to the brim, we headed out. Kellie and I followed Dad, and we travelers drove to LA along the historic Route 66. That was Dad's idea. He promised that driving the famous 2,400-mile road would be fun.

There we were. A little caravan of travelers. Nomads. Gypsies. And I was thrilled! I was moving!

Neither Kellie nor I had ever driven across the country before. We were both fascinated by the varied terrains in different states. The flat plains and rolling hills in Illinois, Missouri, and Oklahoma. The long stretches of arid deserts in New Mexico and Arizona, where the stars looked so close to earth that you could reach up and touch them. I had never seen a sky so wide and open before. When we passed through cities, we noticed how the lights from buildings obscured the stars.

Throughout our road trip, Kellie and I listened to the radio and played silly games like I spy. We drank coffee and sodas from gas stations. When we got hungry, we stopped at convenience stores for snacks. In our car, we munched on granola bars and apples and Cheetos. Kellie and I didn't want to waste much time along the way. We wanted to get to LA as fast as possible.

Dad was in a positive mood. I believed the trip was good for him too. Daniel kept him laughing, and the farther west we drove, the more optimistic he seemed.

I could barely sit still in the driver's seat; I felt such wanderlust. I was going on a journey to find a new persona. A new identity. *Could I do this? Was my wanderlust foolish like Dad had said?*

But still I knew I needed to follow where it led. Instead of simply running to escape my world of pain in Indianapolis, I was racing toward a new beginning and consciousness that would change my life forever.

Dad wanted this road trip to be a fun adventure, so he suggested that we detour to the Grand Canyon. Entering the national park, we drove down a long stretch of road through a forest until we got to the canyon. Then he motioned for us to pull over and stop in the parking lot.

"Oh my God! Oh my God!" Kellie exclaimed. "I can't believe I'm at the Grand Canyon."

"Me too," I said.

When we got out of our vehicles, we took a few steps forward, and there it was. A big opening in the earth. Like an alien planet had just dropped from space into the ground. The *huge*, otherworldly Grand Canyon! Kellie and I could barely contain ourselves. We wanted to go hiking, but Dad reminded us that it would take too much time.

"You girls can always come back for a proper visit someday."

"I will," I told him. "Dad, thank you for bringing us here. It's so beautiful."

"Yes, thank you, Mr. Nick," said Kellie.

"It's something else, isn't it?" he said.

"Beautiful." That was the only word I could think of as I envisioned all those high-desert colors on a canvas.

Dad spread out a blanket on the grass, and we all sat on the ground, eating sandwiches we'd picked up on the way as we looked out in amazement over the landscape. We oohed and aahed while Kellie and Daniel both snapped photos.

It was a mixture of ancient roughness and absolute beauty: rugged canyon walls carved by nature, sandstone flanks, tunneled wind, and a river as thin as a silver ribbon winding through a dusty bed fringed by green trees, red cliffs, and amber-gold rocks and alcoves.

Daniel had been there before. "Every time I come here, it's different. Hiking into it is one thing, floating down the river is another. Every approach reveals something new—another dimension."

"I'd love to take one of those guided raft trips," I said. "I wonder how many miles it covers."

"The canyon is two hundred and seventy-seven miles long, one mile deep, and eighteen miles wide," Daniel replied.

"Wow!" both Kellie and I shouted. We were excited.

It was almost sunset, and the canyon walls displayed fiery crimson and golden hues. As the sun descended behind the rim, softer colors of blue, purple, and green shimmered and vibrated as in a Van Gogh painting in real time. It made me feel that all things were vibrating energy fields in ceaseless motion.

Then the stars began to appear, one by one, in every direction. We gazed up, mesmerized by all those faraway stars lighting the sky above us. I wondered how many people just stopped what they were doing to look up and marvel at the night sky. Not many, I supposed.

For a while, we all sat there mesmerized by the stars. I wondered how many people just stopped what they were doing to look up and marvel at the night sky. Not many, I supposed.

Finally, Dad said it was time to go, and as we headed out, I couldn't help but wonder how Mom would be when I arrived in LA this time. Maybe she would still be stable and would not "go off" like she had so many times before. But a part of me worried, naturally. *Would she tell me that demons were coming? Would she kick me and Kellie out if we brought in items that were, in her opinion, "demonic"?*

There were times on the road trip when I wondered if I had lost my mind, thinking things could work for me in LA. And then there was a part of me that said, *Karena, this is your chance to be with your mom again. To have a close relationship again. It's all going to be OK.* I wanted to believe that part.

I remembered how often I had wanted to die when I lived at home in Indiana. I'd experimented with cutting and taking too many pills and knew it would be so easy to just slip away into a world of nothingness. I wasn't sure there would be a heaven waiting. And I remembered that I had told myself I would hold on to life until I was at least eighteen.

Now, here I was—eighteen. I clung to what the White Tiger had whispered to me during one of my meditations. That I had to leave Indianapolis. That I would die if I did not leave. I had been waiting for this moment.

This was my destiny.

Wanderlust was in my soul.

I was a dreamer.

CHAPTER THIRTY-ONE

Is God Still Watching?

"Inconvenienced"
Song and lyrics by Nick Ivanovich

The simple things we complicate.
A few kind words to relate.
Sometimes feeling good isn't enough.
The willingness to be inconvenienced is love.

Let gratitude refresh the day.
Like morning dew that comes our way.
Let's not waste time in push and shove.
The willingness to be inconvenienced is love.

Eternal child . . .

"Wow! We're in California," I said to Kellie as we sailed down Hollywood Boulevard behind Dad and Daniel. "This is going to be our new home!"

"It's a different world, that's for sure!" said Kellie. "Oh, God, it's so sunny!"

"I still can't get over it. It's so beautiful, and everyone seems so happy!" I laughed with the excitement of a child. I felt like I was seeing sunny California for the first time. "You'll see. You'll love it too."

"You'll be really popular here," said Kellie.

"What do you mean?" I asked.

"You're so tall and beautiful, I bet you'll be discovered by some Hollywood director or something."

I laughed. "Honestly, Kellie, if anyone gets discovered by a Hollywood director, it'll be you. You're so photogenic, and with your long blonde hair, you look like a Cali girl. Trust me, you'll be the one to get discovered."

—

It was just four years ago when I had sat in a high school classroom, worrying about my looks.

Everybody in class thought Kandace was so beautiful. One of my guy friends, Gary, was always saying, "I wish I could get Kandace in my bed!" Even though Gary was just a friend, it made me a little jealous, and I wondered if anyone ever thought that about me. I liked Kandace. She was always nice to me, and I thought she was beautiful too. All the girls thought that. And that's why we were all a little jealous.

Once, at a party, two boys told me that I was cuter than Kandace. That made my night! I welcome any good comments to boost my self-esteem. I don't consider myself beautiful. I was sometimes described as "gangly"—in other words, tall, thin, and awkward. My friends told me that it was a good thing to be called tall and thin, but I just felt the awkward aspects.

—

Thinking about how I worried about my body when I was in high school seemed irrelevant to me now. I had much bigger things to fret about now: money for rent, finding a job, keeping up with the parties and drugs. And finding my way in Cali.

Part of me would always be the eternal child wanting to be loved and nurtured in a way that had been missing for a long time in my life.

But for the moment, I was ignoring all that. To hell with love. It was time to focus on something else.

Powerful forces were quickly energizing the depths of my soul. I didn't fully understand the shift, but I could feel it in my bones. *Perhaps I will finally be happy*, I thought. The idea of living in Los Angeles—in the land of beautiful people and movie stars, sandy beaches and golden sunshine—was exhilarating! *How could I not be happy in such a wonderful place?*

There were a few things I was sure about: In my new adventures in LA, I would not think about all the pain I had experienced growing up in Indianapolis. I would not look for love. I repeated this over and over: *To hell with love!* I would protect myself from being hurt.

I would not let Mom hurt me ever again. We would start over and be friends like many mothers and daughters. I would not let *anyone* hurt me. I would continue to escape my pain in my usual ways but would create a new life on my own. I had a new playground now. In the sunshine and on the beaches. In the ocean waves. There was so much to experience.

Yes, I was going to have a wonderful time. And who knew what life had in store for me? Kellie always wanted to talk about our careers, but I didn't even care about the future, or a career, at this moment. I was just going to enjoy the present because, as far as I knew, that was all I had. I could have inherited my mother's genes and become schizophrenic. I could become mentally ill and lose everything. That was one of my deepest fears: that I would end up like my mother. I couldn't bear that thought. So I took that fear and turned it into a fun and carefree attitude. I simply wouldn't let myself think about the possibility that I could become like her.

Kellie's questions about careers sometimes made me pause. Was it possible I would find a worthwhile career that I loved in this beautiful land? The possibilities were endless, if I let myself dream about them. It didn't matter. *Anything* was better than staying at home and going to Indiana University.

Kellie and I drove straight to my mom's apartment. Mom was at work but had left a key for us under the doormat. She had told me that she would not talk to Dad and would not let him in, so while Kellie and I were unpacking our belongings at Mom's place, Dad and Daniel drove to a motel in Santa Monica where they would stay a couple of days to make sure we were OK.

"I'll bring the rest of your things over tomorrow, when your mom is at work," Dad had said. "After you unpack, call us and we'll come take you girls to dinner."

Kellie and I went in and began unpacking. Mom had said that Kellie and I could share the bedroom, and she would sleep on the living room floor. "I know you girls will want some privacy."

The apartment was still empty. Just a lamp and some blankets and pillows on the floor. There was still no furniture anywhere.

Mom was excited to see us when she came home from work. I was relieved.

"Oh, Karena, you came for me." She hugged me and welcomed Kellie. "I want you girls to make yourself at home."

We made small talk about the drive out.

"Dad and his friend Daniel are staying nearby," I said. "They're coming by to take us to dinner. Do you want to talk to Dad?"

"No." She explained she had a date with a new boyfriend and had plans.

"OK." I didn't want to argue with her.

When Dad and Daniel came to pick us up for dinner, we met them in the parking lot so Mom didn't have to see him. I also didn't want him to be critical of Mom's sparse apartment. At dinner, he asked if everything was OK at Mom's. "Is she being weird?"

"She's fine, Dad," I said. "She's in a very good mood."

Kellie agreed with me. "She seems very nice, Mr. Nick."

"I'm glad to hear that," Dad said. "Karena, do you think she'd talk to me if I came over for a visit?"

"She said she didn't want to talk to you," I said. "I'm sorry. Maybe after some time . . ."

"Sure," he said. Truth was, Dad was over it. He had been since he had flown to California to convince Mom to return home and she'd refused to see him.

Dad and Daniel unloaded the U-Haul for us the next day when mom wasn't home, including twin mattresses we had brought from

Indiana. We put mine on one side of the room and Kellie's on the other side. I also had brought a chair from Indiana, and we used a cardboard box as a side table for Mom's lamp.

After a few days in LA, it was time for Dad and Daniel to return to Indianapolis. It was sad seeing Dad go, but at the same time, I was ready to begin my new life.

"Stay in touch, Karena," Dad said with tears in his eyes. "You know your mother isn't well, so just be careful."

"Of course." I hugged him. "Thanks, Dad, for everything."

"Be safe," he said. "And be happy."

I nodded bravely.

He told me and Kellie to look out for one another, and we said we would.

"I'm just a phone call away," he said.

"I know. Dad, I'm eighteen now. I'll be fine."

Dad tried not to cry.

I tried not to cry.

But there were tears.

Lots of tears.

—

I was eager to put the past behind me. To put Indiana behind me. To put behind me all those moments of riding in a car with Rachel and Dad late at night, looking for Mom and then finding her homeless in a park somewhere.

This escape from those harrowing moments seemed like bliss.

Escape from pain had always been alluring to me.

I should have known that one can't really escape their pain and loneliness by moving across the country. But at eighteen, I thought that I was wise and knowledgeable about life. I had conquered vampires and had emerged powerful. And while I had done these things and taken care of myself for a long time, there was still that eternal child inside me that wanted and needed a mother's love. That child *would never go away* unless I could love myself enough that it didn't matter in the end.

I was still young and naive about trauma, abandonment, and its long-lasting effects on the body, heart, and soul. I did not know that there would always be vampires to slay.

CHAPTER THIRTY-TWO

The Explorer in a New Home

"Compelled by Love"
Song and lyrics by Nick Ivanovich

I may be humbled and left standing in the cold.
My heart shattered and shards driven into my
   soul.
But love gets through the broken edges of the
   heart.
Bringing completeness to who we are.

The flaw...

It was 1999. Everyone was talking about the Y2K bug. People were panicking about a potential flaw in computer systems the world over that would cause utter havoc when the calendar turned from December 31, 1999 to January 1, 2000. But despite weeks and months of worry over Y2K, nothing happened on January 1, 2000. There was a flaw in my own life—in my mindset, though. In my personal world, 1999 meant living in a new state and a new home, but I somehow thought I could continue my wild partying lifestyle and leave all my problems behind in Indiana.

After Dad and Daniel went back home, Kellie and I tried to make a home out of Mom's place. She lived in the heart of Hollywood on Orange Drive. The complex's apartments were clustered around a courtyard with a pool and, from what I could tell, were mostly inhabited by struggling writers and actors. It seemed like everyone carried a notebook with them as they sat in the courtyard, either writing scripts or perusing newspapers and magazines for jobs. They were all dreamers. Creatives. I found that appealing.

But inside Mom's place, it was bare bones.

Kellie and I scrubbed the apartment and tried to decorate it the best we could. We even sponge-painted the living room walls. Mom let me choose the colors, and I selected a gorgeous dark maroon with gold and black accents. The three of us painted together, laughing as we got paint in our hair and all over ourselves. It was so much fun that I felt like a little girl again, recalling how Mom and I had painted our bedroom walls in Indiana.

Oh, Mom, it's so good to have you back. Where have you been for so long? I ached for more times like that with her.

We covered a cardboard box we'd found in the dumpster with scarves, then set candles on it. We bought deli meat and bread at the grocery store, and at night, when Kellie and I were not out partying, we'd light candles and eat sandwiches for dinner. If Mom was home, she'd sit with us and talk about her work. Everything appeared as normal as it could be.

As I was going through my personal things one night, I found a note that my sister Rachel had inserted into one of my shoes.

> *Sissy, I wish I could be out there with you. I wish I could look out for you, so you do not get hurt. Always remember I love you. I wish all happy things for you!*
> *Write me!*
> *Rachel, your Sasha*

It warmed my heart to find this little message. Rachel and I didn't talk all that often, but she was my sister and I loved her. The note tethered me to home, my childhood, my roots, and to her and the life that she and I had always wanted with our mom.

I became an explorer in my new land and established some routines in the City of Angels. Kellie and I spent hours and hours on the beaches of LA, stretching from Malibu to the South Bay of Manhattan Beach. I was especially drawn to the South Bay community. It was laid-back and a haven for outdoorsy folks, tourists, and young families alike. From a beachside perch, we'd watch the surfers, volleyball players, and bikers. Kellie and I practically lived on the beach at Santa Monica, we were there so much.

After my first visit, I'd stayed in touch with Skye. While working and saving money for my move, we had written letters to each other. When I moved out, I contacted him. "I'm here! I'm all moved in and now living here!"

For a while, we spent a lot of time together. Meanwhile, Kellie met a surfer named Harold and ended up staying with him mostly. Skye and I partied with them in the evenings.

About a month after our move, Kellie decided to return to Indianapolis. She came from a wealthy family and had quickly realized she preferred the comforts of living back home. I didn't mind being on my own. I had Skye to keep me company, and I knew I could make new friends.

When Skye and I inevitably broke up, my friend Graham came out to visit. Although we'd kissed when he'd given me Ecstasy and cocaine for the first time, he was now one of my best friends. His older brother lived in Orange County, about an hour south of LA, so that gave Graham an excuse to come visit. He would sleep on the floor with me at Mom's when he wasn't in Orange County with his brother.

In LA, Graham earned extra money as a DJ at raves and talked about moving out here permanently. It wasn't long before we were together. I was crazy about him. I thought he loved me too. We had known each other for such a long time, I thought he was truthful with me.

What I didn't know was that he was also dating a girl back in Indy. In the end, he decided to return home to be with her. He broke my heart.

I reminded myself, once again, that I had to give up on love. It was too painful. Loving people who didn't love me back was a serious flaw of mine. Trusting people who betrayed me reminded me how risky it was to feel. After all, I had my drugs. They would not break my heart.

Kellie was gone.

Skye was gone.

Graham was gone.

I found a job in a boutique on Rodeo Drive in Beverly Hills. But I didn't particularly like that job or the vibe of Beverly Hills, so I looked around and was able to get a better job in a dress shop called Planet Funk in Santa Monica, on the Promenade. It was fun, and I met two new girlfriends, Stella and Cecilia, who were ardent partiers and loved raves and the Hollywood scene.

The raves in California were mostly in dilapidated abandoned downtown buildings and old churches and warehouses. I spent most of my time at those parties when I wasn't working.

All I cared about was my next drug connection. My next party. My next rave.

At the same time, I was enamored with the waves on the beaches of my new home. I was ecstatic about the golden sun in California and the warm, sandy beaches at sunrise. Going to the beach and jumping in and frolicking in the ocean waves was a favorite thing to do in the early morning after a party.

When lying on the beach late one night after I'd been in LA for a while, high and happy, I reminded myself that, at that moment, under the same moon and stars, it was cold back in Indiana with the onset of autumn. There would be moonlit skies and chilly winds whipping through the streets. There would be thick layers of red and yellow fallen leaves from maples, oaks, and ash. Gusts of wind would send the leaves fluttering through the air. Autumn was pretty at times back East, but there was no warmth in the air. For me, there were only lonely memories, pain, and heartache. I remembered how it would turn a midnight dark so early in the evenings during autumn and into winter, and how the tree limbs became haunting shadows that sometimes whispered warnings of vampires and evil.

No, thank you. I did not want to go back to Indiana.

I held so much hope in my heart for my new life, my new home, my California.

And things were mostly OK with Mom.

But I held my breath . . . waiting.

CHAPTER THIRTY-THREE

The Intruder

"Drought"
Song and lyrics by Nick Ivanovich

Learning to weather the storm.
Life has its seasons to mourn.
Crying till the tears run dry.
Dust is filling up the sky.

Make every drop count through the drought.
Quenching the craving of a heart that thirsts.

Seems that life has its cycles
And we've had our share of trials.
I love that Southern California sunshine.
But it doesn't rain for quite some time.

All that is green is turning brown.
Parched by the desert sun
I'm praying for rain to come down.

The nemesis . . .

There was a time when my heart was still open and innocent. Before betrayals and abandonment and intruders.

Now, there was a new nemesis in my world. There was an intruder. And it wasn't Satan.

When Kellie moved back to Indianapolis, I went to a secondhand shop and bought some things to dress up my bedroom. When I lit a candle and turned the lamp on at night, I loved how the soft light made the apartment feel cozier. I would imagine that I was staying in a luxury boutique hotel somewhere in France, and that tomorrow I would meet a new lover named Pierre. My imagination created lovely moments for me even though I was living in a tiny one-bedroom apartment in a seedy area in Hollywood.

Mom was nice at times. She thought my room looked pretty, too, but didn't take any steps in brightening up the apartment. She kept her clothes in a heap in the closet, and her only reading material was the Bible.

Mom and I didn't have any additional paint parties, but she and I got along fairly well during this time. She worked a lot, and I worked and partied, so we didn't see each other much.

I noticed that Mom had been reading her Bible more these days. Flashbacks of living at home and listening to her preaching rushed back to me. I knew this was dangerous territory. Around this time, Mom met a homeless man named John. John was tall, about six foot seven, and from Alaska. Stocky with broad shoulders, dark skin, and thick black hair, he could have been handsome, but his eyes were always bloodshot and his teeth were badly in need of cleaning. Mom said that he had been homeless for years and it was her divine mission to help him.

John turned out to be a severe alcoholic, and when he drank, which was most of the time, he became so belligerent and angry.

Both Mom and John were in their forties; this time could have been the prime of their lives. Mom was doing well at work. But little by little, I saw that her delusions about religion were returning. She told me that I wasn't allowed to bring anything into the apartment with an image on it, just as she'd done back in Indiana. In fact, one time, she found a magazine that I had brought home that had a picture of a

Hollywood actress on the front cover, so she kicked me out for a bit. I had to stay at Graham's brother's home in Orange County. Thank God I had him! Even though Graham had broken my heart, his brother and I stayed friends.

I was allowed back when I'd convinced Mom that I would never again bring anything home—not a book, magazine, newspaper, or a hair-care product—with a graven image on it.

Another time, my friend Shawna came home with me after a night out at a hip Hollywood club. We were only eighteen years old, but nobody carded us back then. And if they did, I had a fake ID. We got in everywhere we went.

Mom stopped us at the door and said, "Your friend can't come in, Karena."

"Why not?" I asked, shocked. "Shawna and I work together, Mom."

"She's not welcome here." Her jaw was clenched.

"What are you talking about?"

Mom clutched the Bible in her hands. "She's the devil, Karena."

"No, Mom, she's my friend. A coworker."

I glanced at Shawna. She shrugged her shoulders as if to say, "No big deal."

I looked closely at Mom's face. She had tied her hair back in a ponytail, which exaggerated her taut expression. And her eyes were wild and a strange, washed-out watercolor blue. I realized she must have stopped taking her meds, and she would probably get worse. Memories of her leaving us flashed through my mind. That pain was still too raw to deal with.

"She's the devil," Mom repeated.

I silently screamed, *But what about John? The guy who beats you? Isn't he the devil?* But I didn't mention John.

I turned to Shawna. I was deeply embarrassed. I had not told her the truth about my mom. "I'm sorry, Shawna. C'mon, let's go. Mom's not being herself today."

Shawna didn't question me, but later, I told her the story. I seldom liked to share Mom's history with any of my new friends. It was too depressing, too embarrassing. Plus, I hadn't forgotten how I had lost several good friends in high school when they learned that Mom was schizophrenic. I didn't want this to happen to me in LA.

I was now on the lookout for more of Mom's delusions. I had hoped that all this strange behavior was behind us, but you can't just run away from your problems. And I should have known that Mom would not keep taking the Haldol. Whenever she was stable on the drug, she said that it robbed her of her creativity. *And your delusions,* I thought.

John stayed at the apartment most of the time while he and Mom were together. I assumed that when he left, he was roaming the streets with his homeless friends to get money for booze.

Meanwhile, I was learning about the disease of alcoholism. That it is just as sly and seductive as drug addiction. John was the last person in the world that Mom needed around her.

One time, John had been in the bathroom, taking a bath, for what seemed like an hour.

"Mom," I said, "what's John doing in the bathroom for so long?"

"He's taking a bath," she said. She stood in the kitchenette, making a sandwich.

I didn't believe it. He was in there forever. When he came out, he smiled like he had a secret.

Later, when I went in the bathroom to brush my teeth, I grabbed the bottle of Listerine to gargle, and it was empty. I walked out and threw the empty bottle at him. "Get out!" I screamed. "You drank all the Listerine to get drunk!"

"What are you talking about, Karena?" Mom asked.

"He's been in the bathroom guzzling Listerine because he's an alcoholic!" I yelled.

"That's not true," John lied.

"It's totally true, and you know it." I was livid.

"Now, Karena, if he said he didn't drink it, then he didn't drink it."

I looked at her like she was an idiot. There was no way I'd convince her otherwise. I finally just let it go.

John often hit Mom in the face or elsewhere on her body. When he hit her, I would attack him and punch his arms and stomach. He just pushed me away and laughed and then pinched my arms hard, often leaving bruises.

I kept quiet about everything that was happening in the apartment when I talked to Dad and even Rachel. I didn't want Dad to tell me that

I had to come home to Indiana. I knew it would worry him, and I just thought it was best to avoid that. For the moment.

Mom never really stood up for herself, and she didn't stand up for me. I had taken on the role of being her protector and knew that I would have to take care of us both somehow.

—

What was that? My ears pricked up, and I tensed, my eyes desperately searching the darkness. It was the middle of the night. Mom and John usually slept on the living room floor under a blanket, but earlier that night, they'd had a fight and he was gone. She'd gone to sleep early. But footsteps moved noisily across the room.

Who's there?

My bedroom door creaked open. My heart leapt into my throat. *Could they hear me breathing?*

Something cold and metallic pressed against my forehead.

Shit! Someone was holding a gun to my head, and a flashlight beamed into my eyes.

I blinked.

What the fuck?

"What's going on?" I asked, my teeth chattering.

"Don't move," the voice said. "I'm Officer Ragsdale, and this is Officer Hasselback. We're with the LAPD. We received a phone call that there's been a murder."

I breathed a sigh of relief that it wasn't an intruder.

A murder?

As I sat up, Mom came running into my bedroom in her pajamas. "What's happening?" The policemen had rushed right past Mom, who had been curled up in the corner of the living room. They must have thought that she was nothing more than a pile of blankets on the floor.

"A man called and said there had been a murder at this address."

"No, that's not right. We're fine," Mom said.

"What man called you?" I asked. I pulled the blanket up to my neck, realizing I was wearing a flimsy nightgown.

"He didn't give his name. It was from a pay phone nearby."

"It must have been John," I said.

"Who's John?" one of the cops asked.

"He lives here." Mom's voice was flat.

They saw the bruises on Mom's arms and asked her about them.

"John . . . the guy who lives with me . . . *accidentally* hit me," she said.

"Do you want to press charges?" one officer asked.

"No," she said. "He was drunk at the time, but when he's sober, he's fine."

"Ma'am, are you sure you don't want to press charges? This is seldom a onetime thing."

"Mom, you should!" I yelled at her.

She shook her head. "No, Karena, I'm all right. And we don't know for sure if it was John who called the police. Maybe he thought he was protecting us."

"No, Mom. He wanted to scare us."

"What about you, miss?" The cop doing all the talking looked directly at me. "Has he beaten you?"

"No, not really," I said. "He has pinched me and pushed me a few times, but that's it."

I didn't want to show them my bruises.

The police officers took photos of Mom's bruises that night as evidence in case anything happened to us in the future.

Finally, the cops left but cautioned us to be careful and stay safe.

We found out later that it *was* John who'd made the call to the police. After their fight, he called the cops to get back at us. It was also possible that he had planned to hurt us and was letting the cops know about it in advance. He was as unpredictable as my mom. But also violent.

Much to my horror, Mom eventually made up with John. This was typical. Since the divorce, she'd often had boyfriends who treated her badly. Neither she nor John ever mentioned that night again. It was as if it had never happened.

Three months after I had moved in with Mom, I came home from my job and saw packed duffle bags in the living room. Mom and John were waiting for me.

"Karena, will you take us to the Greyhound station?"

"Where are you going, Mom?" I heard the slight panic in my voice.

"God told me that I have to go on a journey, and John wants to come with me."

"John's going with you?" I swallowed hard.

"Yes, we're going to get married first and then go on our journey." She smiled like this was the greatest thing in the world.

"Karena, this is a new adventure for me and your mother," John finally spoke up.

How could Mom prefer an alcoholic like John to my father, who had been so dedicated to our family, rescuing her time after time?

My heart raced as a spatter of memories flashed through my mind—memories that hurt so much, my bones ached.

Would Mom leave me one last time, and I'd never see her again? Was this the end of our relationship?

With a wild look in her eyes, Mom just sat there next to John on the newly painted rickety chairs that I had found in a dumpster to go with the cardboard-box table.

Wasn't she sad about leaving me, or worried about me at all? If she was, she showed no emotion about abandoning me in the middle of Hollywood with an apartment I couldn't afford.

"But, Mom, you told me to come to California," I persisted. "You said that we could start over with our relationship and have a new beginning."

"You were going to come out anyway," Mom said.

"I know, but I thought it would be fun to be with you."

"Karena, this is something God wants me to do." She pointed to the Bible that she'd set on top of her duffle bag. "This is the way I keep the devil away. It's not my choice, really."

"But, Mom—"

"So, can you drive us to the bus station?" Mom folded and unfolded her hands.

"You don't want to take *your* car?" I asked.

"You can have the car." Mom's voice was monotone. "I want to be free of all possessions that I have in Los Angeles. I'm only taking the few clothes I have."

Oh, Mom, where have you gone?

I knew there was no use in arguing. "What about the apartment?"

"You can have that too."

"But, Mom?" I attempted one more plea. "What about your job? You've been doing so well."

"Karena, this is my mission. I've saved up some money from my job, and I have to do this. It's my *calling*."

"Linda and I will be fine," John said. "It will be an adventure for us."

I wanted to punch him in the face. I was sure that he did not believe one word of hers about Satan or any mission. He was just using Mom.

"And what about me, Mom, will *I* be fine?"

"Yes, you'll be fine. You have your job and friends."

I had no choice. I finally relented and drove them to the Greyhound station. I hugged Mom goodbye and told her to please call, write, and keep in touch. I didn't hug John. I blamed him for taking her away from me once again. Of course, it wasn't his fault. He was just a crutch. This was her ticket to freedom and a way to avoid being responsible in any way for me, her daughter. And Mom was *his* ticket to anywhere he wanted to go.

I stood outside and watched them get on the bus. They moved down the aisle and sat down in a seat in the back. Mom looked briefly out the window at me, and I raised my hand to wave. She nodded but didn't smile.

As the bus pulled away, my heart broke again into a thousand pieces. I sobbed. I didn't think I would ever see my mother again. *This was the end.*

At the same time, a feeling of freedom swelled up inside me. *Freedom!*

The tears stopped. My nemesis was gone.

The intruder was gone.

CHAPTER THIRTY-FOUR

Mega-Big Stars at Hollywood Parties

"Safe Place"
Song and lyrics by Nick Ivanovich

The fist of life and its busted-up mess.
Cleanup takes time, no need to stress.
I was resting on a bench at a quiet café
When I caught a scent of sweet air blowing my
    way.

I found a safe place, for my broken heart.
I found a safe place, for my broken heart.

We engaged in conversation that would last.
Her light was shining into my darkness.
We ordered up some tea and watched the sunset.
The unspoken pain craves to connect.

Several years have passed since then.
Know the miracle is in the breaking.
Feeling more authentic through it all.
How grace keeps catching my fall.

Independence...

It was extravagant to have two cars, my mom's purple Nissan Sentra and my own Acura. I drove her car after she left until it was eventually repossessed by the automobile dealership. I didn't need it anyway.

I was free. An eighteen-year-old woman on my own in Hollywood. *Independent.* My own person. This was a time to start over. And I was thrilled. That's actually when all the fun began. When I could finally breathe and just enjoy life. I had my own apartment and did not have to worry about Mom's approval or disapproval.

Shawna moved in with me after Mom left, and after a few months, we moved into a two-bedroom apartment off Hollywood Boulevard. We both worked at the Planet Funk dress shop, and when we were off work, we hung out at the beach.

I also had a gym membership where I could work out, and I met Tony, a guy who was very well connected in Hollywood. He took us to a club called Guy's on Monday nights. You had to be a celebrity or know someone to get in. I felt privileged to have that access to Hollywood.

Tony introduced me and Shawna to the whole Hollywood scene, and after that, I didn't do raves anymore. I had moved on and loved it. We would go to clubs and parties, and after the clubs closed, we'd go to crack houses, some of which were in mansions in the Hollywood Hills or in the ghettos. We had a special knock to use on the front door, and someone would open a little window, ask for the password, and then let us in.

My intention was to party as much as possible; escape through cocaine, Ecstasy, and any other drug available; and forget about Mom. It was a repeat in many ways of my life in Indiana, but this time, I had the beach and beautiful weather, and it felt luxurious. And I had movie stars. Lots and lots of movie stars. Everywhere you looked, there were stars and wannabe stars. People continually asked me if I was trying to make it in the movies, or if I was an actor, a model, or a screenwriter. I said no and no and no. I was simply an Indiana girl who loved the beach. I doubted that they believed me.

I found ways to do drugs from night into morning on repeat. While waiting on customers at Planet Funk, I'd often escape to the bathroom to inhale a few lines of coke, and then I'd greet customers with a big smile, rambling on and on about the clothes and prices. The coke made me feel like Miss Personality and gave me self-confidence.

—

Tony told me and Shawna about a party at an exclusive estate in the Hollywood Hills. It wasn't unusual for us to meet Hollywood actors at parties, but when we drove up to this estate and then entered a ball-room with a winding staircase, there were stars everywhere.

I kept thinking: *Is this for real? Am I really partying with Hollywood stars?*

Champagne flowed, and servers with trays of food made their way through the crowds. Cocaine lined the glass coffee tables, and people were openly snorting as I walked past them. I was not high yet and needed some coke in the worst way.

When I saw Mr. Mega-Big Star #1 walk in, I thought I would faint. Or die. I had been a big fan of his ever since I'd seen his blockbuster movie on the big screen back home and could not believe he was right there. He was more beautiful in person than in the movies. I wanted to meet him, but I also wanted to make sure I was extra-bubbly. As usual, I went to the bathroom and pulled a vial from my purse. I shook some coke onto the glistening marble bathroom counter, chopped the powder with a credit card, rolled up a bill from my wallet, and snorted a line. A couple of young starlets came in and smiled. Everyone was doing coke, so it was no big deal. I just preferred doing it in privacy until I got high. Then it didn't matter. The metal taste of the cocaine dripped down the back of my throat. I was so used to its chemical taste that I barely noticed and didn't mind.

I went back out to where everyone was gathered. The music was blasting throughout the rooms, and I felt confident and self-assured. I sashayed through the space like a model and found Shawna.

"I still have plenty of coke left," I told her. "If you need any, let me know."

"I'm good right now," she said, holding a vodka tonic in her hand.

Mr. Mega-Big Star #1 was at the far end of the room, talking to several wannabe starlets. I made my way toward him, but before I got there, I was sidetracked by gorgeous Mega-Big Star #2.

"Hello there." He smiled big at me. Beautiful brown eyes. Beautiful teeth. I recognized him right away from films he'd been in.

"Oh, hi." I giggled.

"My name's—"

"I know," I said, interrupting him.

"What's your name?"

"Karena. Karena Dawn."

"You're really beautiful, Karena. *Karena Dawn*." He looked at me shyly as if he were just an ordinary guy.

"Thank you."

I just stood there smiling like an idiot. *So much for my bubbly personality*, I thought to myself. I couldn't think of a thing to say.

"Can I get you a drink?" Mega-Big Star #2 asked.

"Sure."

I wondered if he knew I was high. Probably. Everyone was high.

"What would you like?"

"Mmm, I don't know. Surprise me."

"OK. I'll be just a minute."

I waited. I was sure he wouldn't come back, so I made plans to find Mega-Big Star #1. But Mega-Big Star #2 did come back. With a glass of sauvignon blanc.

After we talked a bit about how much I enjoyed Los Angeles, he asked if I'd like to go somewhere quiet where we could be alone and talk, and I thought that sounded nice.

I asked him if he was still in a relationship with Mega-Big Star #3.

"No, we broke up a while ago."

"Oh." I smiled at him. "Then, sure, I'd love to go somewhere quiet. Let me find my friend and tell her."

I hurried across the room and told Shawna I was leaving with Mega-Big Star #2.

"Really?" she asked.

"Yeah, really."

"Oh, wow. OK, I won't wait up." She winked at me.

I smirked at her.

Mega-Big Star #2 took me to a nice, quiet piano bar, and we spent the evening just talking. I really liked him. He was gentlemanly, and we ended up dating for a month or so. He became a friend, we partied, and we slept together at his home. I didn't want to take him to my tiny apartment. It was an easy, fun relationship. But it didn't last. Like so many things in Hollywood, and in life, my time with Mega-Big Star #2 was temporary. Nothing stays the same.

CHAPTER THIRTY-FIVE

I Will Die if I Continue

Abandoned is what you see
And then you judge why I am so very alone
Even though I surround myself with people
Who become vampires of the night with me
Red eyes burning deep behind the laughter.
Let me open my heart and soul
So that you can see what being abandoned
Really does to a human.
At first there is the screaming of the soul
Then the falling into emotions that push and pull
The breaking of the brain itself
And it hurts every day
Until the brain stops yearning for love
Because there is a part of you that will always
    remember
How it feels to be abandoned
By your mother time after time because she
    clearly
Has no idea what love is.

—Karena, age twenty-one

My lover . . .

I'm partying with cocaine and meth like this is my last night on earth, but I think that's just the way my mind avoids thinking about the letdown that will come tomorrow. I don't know where I am, but the music moves me like I'm a puppet on strings, my head mashing so hard my brain is in shutdown mode. There's so much sweat on my skin and not all of it is mine. Tomorrow there will be hell to pay, but tonight the drugs keep on flowing. And I am happy and delirious, and I don't care what happens tomorrow.

—

Time passed quickly. I was so busy with my life, I barely noticed that it had been three years without a word from Mom. I was escaping my inner self. I didn't want to explore the mysteries there. The sadness there. The post-traumatic stress there.

My inner self was still a great mystery. It was pure emptiness. As much as I loved Los Angeles and the lifestyle, I still had not really dealt with the abandonment and trauma of my childhood. Or the fact that drugs were my escape.

I learned from my aunt that Mom and John had moved to Colorado. She ended up kicking him out for a while and moving to Evergreen, about a half hour from Denver. I had been living in Hollywood during this time and worked just about any job I could find to pay my rent. I continually lived in fear, waiting for schizophrenia to take over my life. To consume me with the same paranoia and delusions my mom suffered. *After all, it's in my genes,* I reasoned with myself. I didn't believe in anything, and I especially didn't believe in me. I thought I was doomed to become just like my mother.

I still partied like there was no tomorrow. Only, things began to feel different. My partying got so bad that I eventually realized I was out of control and that I could die from too much meth or coke. I knew several people who had overdosed. I'd party all night, then wake up in a park somewhere with friends. We'd cover our faces with our hands when the sun came up, not even knowing how we got there. I realized that we were the vampires I had dreamed about when I was a child. No longer did I have to hide from red eyes glowing in my bedroom window. I was the one with the red eyes who lurked about the shadows in the darkness at night. I was the one who now had to hide from the sunlight.

But at nighttime, things were glorious, and the drugs took over my life. Cocaine was *my favorite lover.*

—

This lover demands that you submit fully to him. Being away from him for too long is unimaginable. When you are together, the world is made whole. He becomes your everything, every thought, every desire. But in the end, he will kill you.

—

The sunlight burned my eyes.

Could someone please turn off that fucking light?

Dogs were barking.

Will you please shut up?

My head pounded as if someone were driving nails into my skull.

I opened my eyes halfway, barely peeking out at the world. The sun was so goddamned bright. I was lying in the grass in a park alongside Alena, a young woman who partied with me all the time. We had been drugging for three days and three nights. I couldn't remember what day it was or where I was.

I could barely move. My breathing was raw, ragged.

I felt certain I was close to death.

Alena started vomiting next to me. I wanted to vomit too. *No, wait.* I smelled of rot. From the looks of my shorts and the rotten stench on my clothes, I had already vomited. *Shit!*

People were walking their dogs in the park and stared at us with disgusted, judgmental looks.

Go to hell!

I pulled myself up to a sitting position and started scratching my arm. And my stomach. I itched all over. I looked down and saw a rash of scaly red bumps on my arms, elbows, and stomach. *What the hell?* It scared me. *Fuck this shit!* It was hideous.

Alena seemed alarmed too. "Karena, what kind of drugs did you do last night? Where did that rash come from?"

"I don't know," I said. "I'll get it checked out."

Alena looked at her arms and legs, worried that she might have the same kind of reaction. "I don't seem to have any breakouts," she said. "Maybe it's from something you ate."

I nodded and pushed my long hair back from my face.

Mornings like this were not unusual for me and Alena. A sadness would seep into my heart as I started to sober up while the sun glared brighter and brighter. It seemed to be shouting at me: *How long are you going to keep this up, Karena?*

My head would hurt all day long, and I'd stay extremely depressed until my next fix. When you come down from a high, you enter a phase of depression that's unlike anything you've ever experienced before. Darkness. Totally void of hope. Your only thought is about how to get your next fix so you can be happy again.

Later that day, I went home and showered and then visited a free health clinic that wasn't far from my apartment. It was filled with people who looked like they were homeless or addicts. It was sad because I was one of them.

When I finally got in to see a doctor, I showed her my arm and stomach.

"It's psoriasis."

"What's that?" I asked. "I've never had this before."

"It's an autoimmune skin condition. Nothing too serious. Usually caused by stress. What's going on in your life?"

"I'm about to turn twenty-one, and life is extremely stressful. I have a lot of anxiety and depression," I said. "I work several jobs to make ends meet. And I party a lot too."

She nodded. "I can give you a topical ointment that will help with the itching and dry it up, but the best thing you can do is lie out in the sun. This will give you lots of vitamin D. I won't prescribe anything for the anxiety and depression right now, but you could start doing yoga and meditation to help with the stress."

"Will it go away?" I asked.

"It should. But it's important to manage your stress and get lots of sunlight."

"I can do that," I said. "I love the ocean and the beach, and I've done yoga before, and I could start running too."

"Sounds good," she said.

It was a wake-up call. I had to make some major changes for my health.

I took the doctor's advice and started yoga again. I got a part-time job working at the front desk of a yoga center in exchange for a membership. I found the yoga studio just fifteen minutes from my apartment in Hollywood, in the valley on Ventura Boulevard. It was called Angel City Yoga, which resonated with me. I worked there twice a week in the evenings and went to kundalini yoga classes every night. Kundalini yoga involves chanting, singing, breathing exercises, and repetitive poses. It's like a physical form of meditation, and is meant to awaken your Kundalini energy, also called shakti, that resides at the base of your spine. Harnessing this energy through the yoga practice is supposed to help you move past your ego, bringing awareness and peace.

I also started enjoying the beach again. Whenever I wasn't working or doing yoga, I was at the beach, falling in love with the sunshine and the ocean. Thankfully, the psoriasis went away.

Next, I bought every self-help book I could find about managing stress and being drug free. And I started seeing a therapist who charged on a sliding scale. I was trying to build a new life and keep my emotional body intact. But I was a mess. I still wanted to party and wasn't always successful in building this new life.

Dad called regularly, and one day, I broke down.

"What happened, Karena?" His voice was soft, kind.

"Dad." My voice quivered. I bit my lip to keep from crying, but it didn't help.

"Karena, what's wrong?"

I gripped the phone with both hands. "I have to make a change."

"What happened, Karena? Talk to me. I thought you loved California."

"I do, Dad," I said. "I love it here, but . . . well . . ."

"What is it?"

I explained how I had been partying night and day and that it dawned on me how I was quickly on the road to becoming an addict, and perhaps I already was. I could die.

As I said these words to Dad, the thoughts chilled me to the bone. I did not want to end up in rehab. Or worse. I would be miserable there. It would feel like prison. And everyone would think I was a failure. I would feel like a failure. I could not let that happen, but it took me a while to free myself from that vampire consciousness. From draining the life force of my body with drugs. I thought I needed the drugs to have fun and escape the pain. But ultimately I was using the drugs to kill the life force within me. Because if one is going to live, one has to accept the pain. It's part of life, and if you can't embrace the pain and work to resolve it, then how can you understand life's joys?

"Karena, I've always known you did drugs. I've always prayed it was just a phase and that you'd grow out of it."

"I want to change, Dad. I really do. But I'm so afraid that I'll become like Mom. You know . . . the schizophrenia and all . . . and for me, drugs have been my escape. I've thought, well, if I'm going to lose my mind, I may as well enjoy what little time I have left."

"There is one thing I know for sure. You are not your mother. You are not going to become a paranoid schizophrenic. And you are mentally strong and independent. You don't even realize your own strength, Karena. You can do anything you want in life. You have a loving heart, and you're so talented and beautiful—inside and out—I know you can overcome this."

"You think so, Dad?" I sniffled and grabbed a Kleenex.

"I'm proud of you, honey." He was sniffling too. I could tell that he was holding back tears. "And I'm here for you if you need anything."

I told him about the psoriasis and that I was now doing kundalini yoga. Of course, I was still doing drugs too—but I didn't tell him that.

"That's wonderful, Karena. Keep it up. I love you, honey."

"Love you too, Dad."

I hung up the phone and sobbed.

But when I stopped crying, I realized I'd had a small awakening. A crack of light had peeked through in my soul where the vampire darkness had taken hold years ago. I had blocked out love and hidden my pain behind a mask of drugs and sadness for ten years. I had not looked at myself closely in the mirror in those ten years because I didn't want to see the person staring back at me.

Thus began my embrace of health and fitness. It wasn't easy to stop the drugs. People still called me to go out and party with them. And there were times that I did. But I was determined to change. To give up my old lover.

I knew that I had chosen a hard path, but I was determined. I had chosen change. It would take a while. I understood that, and I tried to be gentle with myself.

PART SEVEN

Stronger

CHAPTER THIRTY-SIX

San Diego Triathlon

If you do not know a song
How can you sing?
If you do not lift your feet
How can you dance?
If you do not look at the moon
How can you fall into its glow?
If you do not look
How can you see?
If you do not dream of the future you
How can your dreams come true?

—Karena

Transcendence.

The thing about real change is that it is not linear. There will always be obstacles, detours, paths we had not anticipated. One has to learn to take it one step at a time . . . one moment . . . one day . . . one dream . . . one sunrise at a time.

Every day, I watched the sky as dawn transitioned from pink to the color of blue wildflowers while the ocean shimmered like a thousand diamonds. I would take my walk and run along the beach for miles and miles.

Although I had no direct contact with my mother during this time of my life, I was OK with that. It was important for me to let her go. To stop trying to reconnect, as a little girl would, with a loving mother. That simply was not our relationship, and I had to stop fantasizing about it.

Grammy, Rachel, and Aunt Carol would call me from time to time and give me news about Mom. Through them, I learned that Mom and John had gone to his hometown in Alaska. Evidently, John's mother and grandmother were still there. They told me stories about John getting drunk and being put in jail. Mom got a job in a fish factory and at a coffee shop, but John still didn't work. And then he left and moved to Georgia, and Mom followed him. There, he got arrested for being drunk and God knows what else, and was sent to prison.

Mom never contacted me during any of this. And I was glad.

I was training—physically, mentally, and spiritually—in earnest.

This is when the real change began within me. This is when the transformation began. I was now embracing a life that was healthy, drug free, and empowering.

It was exhilarating.

At my father's urging, I enrolled in Santa Monica College. I truly enjoyed the writing classes and felt renewed. I had been going to therapy and doing meditation, plus reading books by Dr. Wayne W. Dyer, Deepak Chopra, and the poet Henry Wadsworth Longfellow, who wrote: "And the night shall be filled with music, / And the cares, that infest the day, / Shall fold their tents, like the Arabs, / And as silently steal away." I recited the words of this poem over and over in my head, like a mantra, a gentle reminder not to allow the worries of the day to overwhelm. I tried my hardest to live this way.

Therapy also helped me to understand myself better. My childhood had been so painful. In fact, my entire life had been painful. It was important for me to understand how to learn from the pain, make good choices, and continue moving forward. I wanted to have a successful life. I wanted to be happy.

My time was now dedicated to healthy eating, fitness, and running. I began to compete in marathons and triathlons. I had actually completed my first half marathon with my dad when I was only twelve years old. I remembered watching my mom doing Jane Fonda and Kathy Smith home workouts on VHS. I even created a workout video in my living room for one of my first school projects. But I had lost touch with physical fitness and health as I struggled with my mom's illness. After experiencing my rock-bottom moment after nights of partying, I decided to go back to what I loved so many years ago. Movement and physical exercise.

Once I started embracing my health, things got better quickly. My love for fitness as a hobby morphed into my profession, and I began working as a personal trainer and then as a sports and fitness model, which led to work as an on-camera spokesperson for major brands like Oakley, Adidas, and New Balance. I was featured in magazines like *Runner's World*, and on the covers of *Triathlete*, *Shape*, *Women's Health*, and *Self*. I began traveling around the world.

But this wasn't the end-all for me. There was more that I wanted to accomplish in life. I had a bigger mission. I wanted to *give back*. It was important for me to look out for others, especially women. I wanted to empower them and help them to overcome their own weaknesses and to learn how to survive when mental illness affected their families and circles of friends. I wanted to be a mentor for them so they, too, could learn how to live their best lives.

The San Diego Triathlon was my next challenge. I knew how difficult and painful this triathlon would be. How exhausting it would be. But also how exhilarating it would be. It scared me. Could I do it? Fear was my biggest obstacle.

I was so familiar with fear. I had lived with it all my life.

Fear holds us back and closes our minds to possibility. It imprisons us in our comfort zone. But what you come to realize is the more you push those boundaries of what is comfortable and safe—the more you live outside your comfort zone—the less hold fear has. It retreats into the margins. I have learned to do what scares me and have discovered that by doing so, less and less does.

I have also learned that all of us can rewire our brains to overcome fear. It just takes training. You have to commit to the hours of practice and repetition. Whether you are training for a marathon, learning a new language, studying for a test, or traveling somewhere unknown, you are mastering new skills, and all of this is rewiring your brain and helping you master fear itself. So every time I worked out, whether I was running along the beach or doing weight training in the gym, I was rewiring my mindset as well.

In addition, meditation also rewires your brain and helps you stay calm. I had been meditating for a long time. During meditation, you can detach from the mental chatter, the outer noise, and emotional states. So while I was physically training, I was also emotionally and mentally training through meditation. It rewired my brain and changed my thought patterns.

I began training for the San Diego Triathlon with all this in mind. As I got stronger, my body also created more natural mood-enhancing chemicals like serotonin, dopamine, and norepinephrine, which flooded my brain for a couple of hours postexercise. It was thrilling and motivated me even more to continue my healthy lifestyle.

The night before the triathlon, I had to get up at two thirty a.m. and head to San Diego. I dreaded it. The first thing I would have to do was swim in the cold ocean. I tried to keep my mind focused on the thrill of completing a triathlon as I mentally checked off everything on my packing list: swimsuit/wet suit, goggles, swim cap, bicycle, cycling shorts, cycling shoes, water bottle, protein bars, running shoes, music, towel, sunglasses. I was quite sure I had everything I needed.

During the drive, I tried to relax and focus on the moment. I gazed into the dark sky and saw some stars near the crook of the moon.

As the birthplace of the triathlon, and with an ideal climate year-round, San Diego and its surrounding areas are full of awesome triathlon events, so this was an appropriate place for me to experience my first one. For every race I've run, there has never been a question of stopping before the finish line is crossed. I wasn't always good at pacing myself, but I knew how to keep going even when my body was aching and hurting and told me to stop. There was always a reserve somewhere inside me.

I had trained for the San Diego Triathlon by myself. Running. Biking. Swimming. Meditating. Reading. Rewiring my brain.

I was scared but also happy.

Hundreds of athletes had already arrived at Spanish Landing Park by the time I got there, around four a.m. I parked and took the shuttle to the start area. The swim was wet-suit legal, and I carried mine to the swim start, about a mile away from where the shuttle had dropped me off. Most people were struggling with putting on their wet suits, but I had actually given instructional videos on how to do it, so it wasn't as difficult for me as it was for them.

We lined up in our corrals: pros, elites, men in different age brackets, and then the women. Electricity buzzed in the air with people talking, full of anticipation, nerves, and excitement.

As I took my mark, I thought about everything that had come before: how the evil ran after the little girl, determined. I was that little girl . . . I ran away from it, tripping and sprawling . . . And when it caught me, it raged through me with the sound of crushing wind, white-hot in its fierceness, leaving me numb to all. Right then, I said goodbye to the little girl and hello to the strong woman I was becoming.

The water was icy cold when I jumped in, triggering an immediate panic attack in the water. I couldn't breathe, and for a moment, I thought I would die. My yoga training was the only thing that got me through that panic attack. By using various breathing techniques, I calmed myself, lowered my heart rate, and moved on.

As I swam, I focused on keeping my head down and moving forward. *Keep going, Karena,* I told myself. *Keep moving forward.*

Still, my thoughts returned to my past. I was scared of what my memories held—all the times my mom abandoned me, which never seemed to escape me. They were pinpoint needles piercing my skin. I couldn't scream or fight back. I just had to endure the pain.

As I reached the barge on the other end, I was yanked out of the water onto the ramp by a volunteer. I had no idea how long it took me to swim those thirty-nine meters.

From the ramp, we ran about a third of a mile down an asphalt path. By the time I reached my bike, my feet were almost numb, but I managed to get my shoes and helmet on, and I climbed up on my bike and started pedaling hard.

The sadness flowed through my veins and deadened my mind. It was like a poison to my spirit, dulling other emotions until it was the only one that remained. It was as if a black mist had settled upon me and refused to shift, and no matter how bright the day was, I would not be able to feel the sun or hear the birds sing. For in that sadness, the world was lost to me, and I knew of nothing that would bring it back into focus.

I pulled my thoughts back to the bike ride. *Focus, Karena, focus.*

Enjoy. The twelve-to-eighteen-mile bike course was fun as I pedaled along a mountainous path to the Cabrillo National Monument and back. The hills were long enough that I could really increase my speed when I went downhill. As I approached Spanish Landing Park again, I was met with beautiful seaside views and challenging elevation gains. The next transition, to the run, was quick, and my legs felt fairly good, even though they were a bit wobbly. Right out of transition, we ran up a very steep hill, so I had to push through some aches, but I finally made it to the top.

I wanted to scream from memories surfacing. I muffled my sobs. The world turned into a blur, and so did all the sounds. The smells. Painful emotion after painful emotion from my childhood slammed against me before I lost feeling. I thought about loves won and loves lost. Everything inside darkened into nothingness as I continued forward. What I was moving toward was light, freedom, and exhilaration.

The crowd was waving and cheering wildly, and I attempted to soak up the energy. I tried to pay attention to the gathered fans while also getting lost in memories and making plans for my future as the finish line came into sight.

Stone by stone, the wall collapsed. It could not hold and I just broke. The tears pierced the membrane, cleaving muscle, bone, and gut. I felt hollow. Then, suddenly, I crossed the finish line, and my cheering friends and fellow athletes had reached into my hollowness and made me feel whole again. And then from somewhere deep inside, I heard that voice I had quieted for too long: *You already have everything you need right here. We all do. Greatness is in each and every one of us; we only need to get out of its way.*

With that thought, finally, the hardest part of my journey with my mom was done. I knew there would be times when I would encounter my mother in the future. Of course. But I did not have to let her bring me down anymore.

I collapsed on the ground, breathing in deeply. Tears streamed down my face. Tears of joy, release, and happiness.

This was a new me. Karena 2.0. Reinvented. Reborn.

After I don't know how long, I finally stood up, wiped the tears from my eyes, breathed in the fresh air, raised my arms to the sun, and shouted, "OK, world, I'm coming for you! Let's see what else I can do!"

PART EIGHT

Full Circle,
The Sunset

CHAPTER THIRTY-SEVEN

The Tone It Up
Fitness Festival Tour

"Mantra of Love"
Song and lyrics by Nick Ivanovich

I kissed you at the edge of Celery Bog
As the sunshine burned off the morning fog
In the soft ground and moss
Two sycamores were standing
And a blue heron was gliding in for a landing . . .
This moment . . . saved me . . . so relaxed and
    easy . . .
This moment . . . filled with light
Shining with pure delight

Rusty blackbird
Singing along the wooded trail . . .
How much sweet air did we inhale . . .
And the love just keeps pouring out
Need this without a shadow of doubt
This moment . . . saved me . . . so relaxed and
    easy . . .

This moment . . . filled with light
Shining with pure delight
Out in nature . . . life can be so nice
Listen deeper to the quiet voice inside

Red-bellied woodpecker
Hitching along trunks of trees
All the sights and sounds
Flowing through me
This moment . . . saved me . . . so relaxed and
    easy . . .
This moment . . . filled with light
Shining with pure delight

Beautiful.

This moment. This situation. This sunset. The twilight leaned into me. All lavender and pink. Colors fading from salmon to crimson. Behind the cathedral-tall New York buildings, ribbons of periwinkle seep into the horizon.

Bobby was not with me physically, although he was never far from me, not really. While I was on this trip, he was at home in California, taking care of Skunk and looking after my mom. He was my rock. My North Star. And it was because of him that I was where I was on this day, and that Mom was where she was. Balanced. Happy. Her suffering had not been in vain. Nor had mine.

I felt like I had come full circle in just the few months since January 2017, when Bobby and I had moved my mom from the hospital in Seattle—where the doctors had suggested she go into a nursing home—to an apartment in the small town of Idyllwild, California, where she could live on her own and still be cared for.

So much life had happened during those past several months. So much pain. So much change. So much growth. So much love. Now alone, I looked out the window of my hotel room in New York City. Lit candles cast a soft glow across the shadows in my room. It was a quiet time for reflection. It was a sacred moment.

All week, my business partner—the cofounder of our fitness app, Tone It Up, Katrina Scott—and I were featured on television talk shows, joining meetups to get to know some of our favorite New York City Tone It Up gals, and interviewing with magazines like *Self* and *Forbes*. Earlier that evening, we'd met friends over a glass of wine and talked nonstop about our tour.

The next day, after I completed my morning ritual of meditation and coffee, I joined Katrina for our next Tone It Up Fitness Festival Tour event in Brooklyn. Jillian Michaels, the personal trainer for the hit television show *The Biggest Loser*, was also there.

Our tour consisted of fifteen stops in thirty days in key cities throughout the US, where we worked with thousands and thousands of women of all ages.

I was humbled whenever I recalled the moment our business began, when I met Katrina at a gym in California in 2009, and we created the Tone It Up fitness company with $3,000 of our own money. We committed to helping others achieve their optimal fitness and lifestyle, and through this mission, our group grew into a worldwide community of millions of strong, beautiful women.

I'd long ago learned to let go with wild abandon and breathe in the sunsets. I'd shaken off my sorrow through my fitness training and meditation, and Tone It Up was all about helping other women do the same.

Now, here in New York City, signs of life were everywhere. It felt like a testament to everything I had experienced, from my traumatic childhood and turbulent years in LA to the life I'd created for myself: founding Tone It Up, marrying Bobby, helping my mother finally achieve health.

I'd found my footing.
My voice is loud.
Strong.
I am the alchemist.
I have come full circle.

—

"Inhale," I said into my mic. "Exhale."

People forget to breathe.

The sun glittered gold in the early morning on a pier at the Brooklyn Bridge Park, the bridge rising stoically against the Manhattan skyline.

A sea of people stretched from the Tone It Up stage to the East River. Hundreds of ladies with their mats and water bottles, ready to exercise. The event was sold out.

Music by DJ Madds pumped up the energy. A nearby Braid Bar offered hair braiding. At these fitness festivals, Tone It Up also featured a merchandise tent, beauty salons, and the Core Intention Tent. We had tables set up for back massages, as well as photo booths, sample protein drinks and kombucha, food trucks, and more. And all the attendees were given a swag bag and a bracelet. It was a true festival.

Our tours featured three workouts, each about a half hour long: CorePower Yoga, cardio by Jillian Michaels, and booty/core work with me and Katrina. Some of the Tone It Up fitness trainers, including Chyna, Stefi, Tori, and Chevy, came with us too.

But the most important part of our Tone It Up Fitness Festivals wasn't the instructors. It was the audience that made each festival a success. The connections among the people committing with one another to becoming better versions of themselves, and the connections with body, soul, and mind. Everyone was welcome: diehards, rock stars, newbies, millennials, and baby boomers.

"C'mon, push! You can do it!" I shouted. *"You can do it!"*

Hundreds of arms were flung high into the sky. Legs kicked. Ponytails flopped back and forth. The women sweated, guzzled water, and had fun. And we were all present in the moment.

Finally, Katrina and I led a cooldown with plenty of stretching, and the main event was over.

By the time Katrina and I headed for the meet and greet at the VIP Lounge, dark clouds had bunched together in the sky and the air had turned cooler. Twilight settled.

The VIP Lounge was decorated with pastel-colored sofas, pillows, and blankets, and we served complimentary rosé. We met attendees and took photos with them.

One of the Tone It Up participants came up to me and asked for a photo.

"Hi, I'm Grace," she said, all smiles. Sweat glistened on her arms.

"Nice to meet you. Have you had a good time?" I asked.

"Honestly, your and Katrina's sculpting class was awesome. From the squats to the dance breaks, that workout was amazing."

"It's rough, I know." I laughed. "I hope the music helped."

Grace nodded. "I mean, one minute, we're struggling to get through a set of leg lifts, and the next second, there's you and Katrina next to us, cheering us on. Pushing us through the workouts with you. It's really motivating."

I smiled at her.

The moment was remarkable.

I was bursting with joy: *I am whole.*

CHAPTER THIRTY-EIGHT

The Hero's Journey

"Love Always Wins"
Song and lyrics by Nick Ivanovich

So many mysteries in the stars above
But you can never escape the reach of love.
'Cause love always wins
Even after the last whisper of the night has been
    silenced.
'Cause love always wins
Even after the final episode of the ravages of life
    and violence.
'Cause love always wins.

Memory.
    And so, it was . . . A low humming sound, constant and rhythmic in its harmony, reverberated from a black hole in the cosmos. This sound, as it had done for billions of years, warbled from the galaxy of stars and created a cadence in the heavens. Vibrational and multi-textured, this cadence rippled as a chant from the higher planes and trickled into the lower worlds to all who could hear it. This was the formation of memory, part of the sound.

—

By the end of our time in Seattle, Bobby and I had decided to take a leap of faith and move my mother to an assisted-living facility, and then to her own apartment in a small town in California, not far from where we lived. There, she had stabilized, and we began rebuilding our fractured relationship. After so many years of pain, we were now both healthy enough to appreciate what we could provide each other and how we were linked.

I had a dream one night about memory. About loved ones, our friends and families, our connections, our DNA, Babushka, Geed, and many of my relatives who have lived before me and moved on to other worlds. It surprised yet comforted me, reminding me how we are all connected and that there's a reason for everything that happens to us.

—

We have been lost to each other for a long time. It has been so long, you probably do not even know my name. Memory tells me, "I am hidden by the thousands of moons that have passed across the sky. It is no one's fault, really."

Memories often become lost after the passing of each new moon. They fade and discolor like old newspaper clippings, and finally turn into dust . . . And unless there is a thread—a bond of love that's anchored by memories—we become lost to one another. And no matter where you live, no matter the city or country, the chain connecting one generation to another is broken if the memories disintegrate.

—

One day, Bobby and I sat with Mom in Idyllwild, California, on the deck of a café, having lunch. I was aware of what Bobby had given me. Mom was aware of what he had given her. He was the rock of strength. The foundation, the connection that glued our lives together.

I was in awe of my mother. Of her strength. It is true, you know. Our mothers build the emotional tapestry of our lives, from one generation to the next, and this tapestry is continually being woven into the lives of our descendants. New experiences are added to the weave while old tears are being mended. And so, it was this way with me and my mother.

At that moment, we were surrounded by tall pines, sweet-smelling cedars, and rocks legendary for climbing. Idyllwild is a charming, artistic village with fewer than four thousand residents, featuring locally owned shops and restaurants. It boasts a homey, community environment that offers hiking and respite from loud city life. Bobby and I ordered salads and grilled fish, and Mom had a pita sandwich. We talked about everyday things like the weather, friends, and family. We laughed, pondered, and chatted about art and happiness, and the future.

The eternal chain connecting loved ones to life has not been lost on humankind. It is in our DNA, generations before us.

At some point in time, we all struggle to find purpose in our life, and other times, we learn that knowing our purpose isn't the struggle. The struggle—any struggle—is the defining moment of our existence.

And these struggles, this emotional pain we carry from the battles waged, make us braver and stronger and more resilient. No one's suffering is in vain. Mom's illness made me stronger. It made me the woman I am today. Memory now celebrates the humanity within me.

From all of this, love is born.

I thought back to when we brought Mom to California from Seattle a few years ago. The changes in her were remarkable. She was now living on her own in Idyllwild, which is perched amid the pine and manzanita trees of the San Jacinto Mountains, between Hemet and Palm Springs. It has no chain stores, just two gas stations, and none of the traffic and smog that plague the cities to the west. Mom was stable and vibrant. She was happy, creating artwork, and enjoying her life. We had all grown. We were friends. And we were family. Our own unique family.

She thrived there. And I thrived because of her.

Without memory, we would all become just a footnote, our story a brief detour between the celebrated chronicles of life, relationships, war and peace. We would all become a grain of sand on the ocean's beach . . . nothing more than a microcosmic speck of gold in a stream of dust. Forever lost behind the thousands of moons that grace the sky. We are so much more than that.

When you practice acceptance and forgiveness in this lifetime, and try to deeply understand another human being and recognize the bond and the DNA shared between a mother and daughter, then you will become an alchemist and find the gold in life.

I recognized that there is a powerful strength inside my mother. I recognize that my drive, courage, and strength come from her. They are simply manifested in a different way. When I was younger, I just thought she was sick and had abandoned me. But she was on earth to teach me how to be strong. I would have never achieved what I have today if my mother had been any different. She taught me to be resilient. Like the women in our family before her.

My mom is the hero in my journey. In my story. And I honor her and love her.

Each of us must navigate our ancestry, the world, and society with all the infinite uniqueness of our family, personalities, individual talents, and proclivities. We must find our place in the beautiful brokenness that is humanity and observe and translate what we discover along the way, because each of us is so much more than our human self. We simply become blinded by humanity when we are on earth.

We must let memory take our hands and lead us through a labyrinth of flowers atop a hillock covered with dense trees. We must meander through deep and remote areas of DNA, where nature procures the delight of abstrusity. There, we will find our ancestors. There, I will find Babushka and Geed, Grammy and Grampa . . . And that is where I will find myself, among all my ancestors who have gone before. My loved ones. Past, present, and future. "We remember you," they tell me. "We love you. You are not forgotten."

And I take joy and comfort in this, as I hope all of you will when you read my story, so you can remember your own story and find the love that's waiting.

EPILOGUE

Dedicated to
Linda Joy Tompkins
1954–2021

"I Want to Sing a Song"
Poem by Rachel Sahaidachny

I want to sing a song—I hear my voice, but no
    words.
In your life, I struggled to know you.
It was hard to love you.
In your death the unknown of you stretched like a
    shadow in front of me.
Kneeling in the dirt of your grave, I heard you.
I heard you say, I'm done with sorrow!
The northern winds blew through the brush and
    trees surrounding me.
You held enough sorrow in this life for every
    other lifetime
To be filled with Joy.

San Diego Hospital
September 2021

Angels.

Angels hovered in the hallways, in the patients' rooms . . . angels, everywhere. Sparkling, twinkling, scattering lights signaled their beings . . . Soft melodies trilled in the air, carrying their songs for life . . . for love . . . for me, for my family, and so it was . . . as always . . . a low humming sound, constant and rhythmic in its harmony, reaching out to beings everywhere.

Death stood close by. "I have a few stops to make before this one," he wrote in the Big Diary of the World. "But not right now. She still has a little more to teach others. But yes, in a little while, her suffering will be over. Not now but soon."

Angels shooed Death away. For the time being.

—

I couldn't do it.

Go on, I told myself. *One more step.*

I sat in the waiting room and wiped away the tears that were streaming down my cheeks. Before I could go into the ICU, I had to dress from head to toe in white coveralls, with paper over my shoes, disposable gloves, and a mask. They were taking extra precautions because of the COVID-19 virus. And only two visitors were allowed at a time. Aunt Carol had already flown in to say goodbye.

Entering a hospital to see my mother was not something new. Especially after I became her caretaker. As a teenager, Rachel and Dad were generally with me. And later, in California, it was just me and Bobby. We'd visit, and then Mom would get better and be released.

But this was different. I wasn't sure that Mom would recover from this.

As I sat in the waiting room, I found myself unable to walk in.

I called my best friend and business partner, Katrina.

"Kat."

"Karena?"

"Kat, I don't think I can face going into my mom's hospital room."

"Karena, you can do this." Her voice was soft. "Your mom needs

you right now, and you are strong. You are one of the strongest people
I know."

"But, Kat—I—I—She's in the ICU, and her doctors told me they
weren't sure how long she had to live. And—"

"I know. But she's alive right now and she wants to see you."

She reminded me that Mom loved me and that I loved her.

"Is Bobby with you?"

"Not this time, but he'll come if I ask him."

"That's good. I'm here for you too, if you need me."

"Thanks, Kat. I'll talk to you soon."

"Love you, Karena."

I breathed in deeply and walked down the hallway to the ICU.

I had been contacted by the physicians at this San Diego hospital
when Mom was brought here five months ago. I had checked on her repeatedly, making sure she was being taken care of. It was not unheard
of for Mom to go to the hospital after she'd lost a lot of blood. She had
been doing quite well in her cabin in the mountain village of Idyllwild
for a while now, painting pictures and enjoying nature. It was during
those good times when it felt as though Mom might remain stable and
be OK. But then, something would happen, and her old illnesses, including the bleeding disorder, would resurface, like now.

Two weeks ago, Mom texted me and asked me to call her.

Her voice was thin and scraggly, like that of an old woman. Much
older than her biological age in the midsixties.

"Karena, they can't stop the bleeding."

Mom's bleeding disease had been diagnosed as HHT, a disorder in
which some blood vessels do not develop properly. It's not always fatal,
but it can shorten a person's life.

Since Mom called, I had talked to her doctors almost every night
about her condition. She was now receiving comfort care and pain
medication.

Just breathe.

I pushed open the door to my mother's room.

I was shocked when I saw her. She had aged a thousand years. Her
arms had dark splotches everywhere from the nurses drawing blood.
They were bare-bones skinny and wrinkly like those of a ninety-year-
old woman. Her stomach was distended, and her hair, gray and wiry.

Mom was hooked up to an IV, and a tube connected to a monitor recorded her heartbeat. Another monitor on her finger checked her pulse.

I wanted to burst into tears, but I held back. I walked over and took her hand.

She opened her eyes, once a bright blue but now dull gray. And she smiled. "Oh, Karena, honey, I'm so glad you're here."

In my sadness, there was no past or future. I was just living moment to moment, the best I could, from the second I woke up into this new reality until my body could do no more and sleep came to rest my weary mind. Each day, I greeted the sun like a climber greeting their rope, fingers holding on fast despite the pain and heartbreak. This was grief.

I think grief came to my mom this way too. I believe the sadness flowed through her veins, as if the world were slipping away from her, and she knew of nothing that could bring it back into focus, although she tried.

For the first three days I was there, and once while Aunt Carol was sitting with us, Mom would have little bursts of energy. *Karena, come sit over here. Carol, can you sit over there? And, Karena, can you get me more water?* Little things like that. Once, she looked at me and said, "Karena, you are so beautiful." She then looked at Aunt Carol and said, "Carol, you used to be beautiful."

Aunt Carol just shrugged her shoulders. "Well, you were beautiful too, Linda."

Mom became focused on regret. I couldn't scream at her. I couldn't blame her anymore. All I could do was let go. I had to move past all the disappointments and tell her I loved her over and over again.

"Mom, please don't regret anything. Everything you did helped me become the person I am today, and I am grateful for that."

She had been in denial all her life. She wouldn't face her physical or mental-health issues. She pretended throughout life that she was fine. But deep down, she knew. She struggled for many years. I have all her old journals, and I know how painful her life had been. The extraordinary thing about all of it was that she was a fighter . . . up until the last moment.

Finally, it was time.

Bobby stood by my side as we said our goodbyes to Mom, along with Aunt Carol and Rachel. We held her cold, tiny hands and together read Psalm 23 to her. "The Lord is my shepherd . . ."

—

SHE'S GONE TO HEAVEN

San Diego Hospital
September 15, 2021
12:33 a.m.
Death and the angels.

Death watched carefully and sighed, "The time has come."

He scooped her up and wrapped her in his arms, gently and lovingly. Tears streamed down his face. This was not an easy job. But he consoled himself, knowing that where he was taking this loving soul was a place of ultimate beauty and happiness, joining her with loved ones who were calling. Death knew that the purpose of Linda Joy Tompkins's life was the struggle in teaching her daughters how to be strong and grow into beautiful individuals. It was the defining role of her existence. Still, he sighed. It was always difficult to take the souls, even though there was so much joy waiting.

Angels gathered close by in an aura of golden light that sparkled like jeweled fractals.

With the greatest of care, Death carried her to the angels and the loved ones who were waiting.

—

White cranes and gulls soared across the clear, crystal blue sky, and the sun shone bright. Ocean waves frolicked back and forth in the Pacific. Bobby and I were staying at the Lodge at Torrey Pines, overlooking the ocean.

"Mom has gone to heaven to be with the angels." My voice was small, quiet.

"I know." Bobby took my hand. "She is free now."

I sighed. I was grateful that Mom was now pain free and hopefully happy, but grief had carved unbearable pain and sorrow into my soul. It would take time to reassemble the broken parts of myself.

I knew now that this was actually just the beginning of my healing journey.

LESSONS I HAVE LEARNED
THAT MIGHT HELP YOU

Caretaker: Being a caretaker is learning to let love take over. It's beautiful and painful at the same time. Just breathe. Know that you are enough.

Empathic introvert: It's not easy to maneuver in this world if you're an empathic introvert. We are very sensitive individuals who can feel and experience the emotions of people close to us. And we often feel overstimulated by mobs of people and loud sounds. This trait also makes it difficult to be a caretaker. We absorb the emotions and feelings of the people we care for, and that's challenging. Accept who you are. Know that if you're an empathic introvert, you are probably one of the most creative people in the world. Know that your capacity to love is bigger than the world itself. And you do not have to be like the extroverts, who actually gain energy by being around many people. We introverts are the creators: the artists, the writers, the readers, the musicians. We empathic introverts are the protectors of history and dreams. We are the keepers of memories.

Acceptance: Can you work toward acceptance in your relationships? Accepting that my relationship with my mother would never be what I wanted or was hoping for was a step toward healing. I work on this every single day.

Parentification: This is when a child takes on the parenting role in their relationship with a parent or sibling. If you have experienced this, name it so you can work with it. I have been the parent in my and my mom's relationship. These childhood experiences often led to adult feelings of anger, anxiety, poor self-esteem, and mistrust in peer and romantic relationships. Parentified children also often continue the role of caretaker into adulthood, which is what happened with me. But

I decided to use this as a strength. Mom was almost like my child later on, and I learned to love her in that way. I had to release my hopes and expectations of Mom actually behaving like a mother usually would.

Addiction: I have learned that not knowing how to be authentic in my teens and early twenties led me to addiction and hiding parts of myself from the world. If you are experiencing addiction, there are numerous organizations and therapists who can help.

Loving relationships: Learning how to trust and love someone romantically, and letting that person love you, will make you a stronger, more empowered person. At one point, I had sworn off all romantic relationships. I'm happy I learned how to trust and love again. And yes, it might take therapy to help you learn this, but it's possible. You, too, can have a loving relationship in your life.

Worthiness and value: Learn to value yourself. To know beyond a shadow of a doubt that you are worthy of the best. I have, by focusing on fitness, meditation, yoga, and therapy. All of these have helped me grow to be the person I am today. And reiterating one of my earlier lessons, I know that as an empathic introvert, I am worthy and valuable. And knowing this makes me braver than I ever imagined.

Surrender: Be open to surrendering to others, knowing that it's OK if you cannot do it all. You cannot take care of everything. You cannot take care of everyone in your life or in the world. Know when to ask for help. We all need help in this world, and there are others who will help if you just ask.

Imperfections: Love your imperfections. People are so hard on themselves. Please, don't be. We all have problems and dragons to slay. We all have our to-do lists and believe we're failing if we do not get everything done. It's OK if you're not perfect. That's what makes you interesting and beautiful.

The small stuff: Don't sweat it. The criticism someone might have made when you did or said something. The pounds you may have gained over the holidays. The fact that you got passed over for a job you really wanted. It's all small stuff when you think about it. Look inside your heart and know what truly matters.

Forgiveness: Hate will eat you alive. It will destroy you. Forgive others even when they have been horrible to you. I have learned to forgive my mother for being mentally ill with paranoid schizophrenia. I have learned that everything in my life has been designed in a perfect way for me to achieve my very best. Her illness helped me to evolve and grow, and ultimately, I learned how to trust again.

Setting boundaries: I believe people should forgive others for their indiscretions and harmful actions. I also believe it's important to set boundaries. Being loving does not mean letting people walk all over you. If someone tries to harm you emotionally or physically, cut the ties. You do not deserve to be treated badly by anyone. I had to figure out how to set boundaries with my mother. She had a tendency to manipulate me, and I had to learn how to say, *No, this is not acceptable.*

Releasing guilt and shame: We all feel guilty sometimes, and then we spend a lot of time feeling shameful about whatever it is that we did. I felt very guilty about doing drugs and making poor choices. I had to learn how to release that guilt and shame and not let it define me. And I have learned that it's OK to speak about the "dirty" stuff in our lives. The embarrassing stuff.

Grief as a teacher: I have learned how to allow grief to be my teacher. I have learned to let myself cry and feel all the heartbreak and disappointments from my mother and others. It has taught me that once you're past the grief, you can open the door to more love. For, in the end, life is ultimately about love. There is nothing else.

Love: I have learned that people are brought into our lives for a reason. Struggles, hardships, and disappointments are all designed to help us become stronger, to grow. I have learned that my mother gave me the greatest gift on earth. Because of who she was, I am a successful, happy woman today.

Action step: Readers and friends, make a list of things you have learned in your life and even things you are working on. Keep a notebook on hand and write down lessons as you identify them. This is healing. Find the love.

Finally, my darlings, be inspired by this book and embark on your own journey of self-awareness and growth. And know and say this with me:

I am enough.

Let me repeat that.

I. Am. Enough.

ABOUT THE AUTHOR

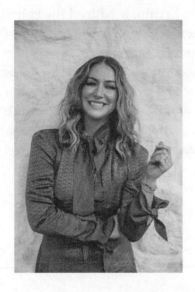

Karena Dawn is an entrepreneur, trainer, bestselling author, and co-founder of Tone It Up, the leading fitness and lifestyle community for women. Her lifelong passion for fitness, mindfulness, and spiritual empowerment has made her a leader in the wellness space. Born and raised in Indiana and currently living in Austin, Texas, by way of California, Dawn began cultivating her spiritual practice from a young age. Meditation and movement transformed her life and helped her overcome a dark period of depression and substance abuse. Since then, she has practiced daily meditation and followed The Seven Spiritual Laws of Success for more than ten years. She is honored to speak about The Seven Spiritual Laws and how to apply them to your everyday life.

As the cofounder of Tone It Up, Dawn empowers women around the world. Through workouts, nutrition products, and community connection, Tone It Up helps women live their healthiest and happiest lives. Most recently, Dawn created Toned Body, Toned Mind, a holistic program in the Tone It Up app that combines yoga, meditation, and self-care practices and includes many teachings she learned while studying meditation at The Chopra Center. She is the coauthor of *Tone It Up: Balanced and Beautiful* and the *New York Times* bestselling book *Tone It Up: 28 Days to Fit, Fierce and Fabulous.*

Dawn has been featured in *Forbes* for creating a "fitness empire" and on the Create & Cultivate 100 List honoring women who are masters in their field. She has also headlined the POPSUGAR Play/Ground festival and has been a keynote speaker at the Power Up Women's Leadership Conference.

As a passionate advocate for mental wellness, Dawn is proud to serve on the board of advisors for NAMI (National Alliance on Mental Illness) and is the founder of the mental health nonprofit The Big Silence Foundation, as well as the podcast *The Big Silence.* Through all her work, Dawn is dedicated to helping others feel confident, empowered, and fulfilled.